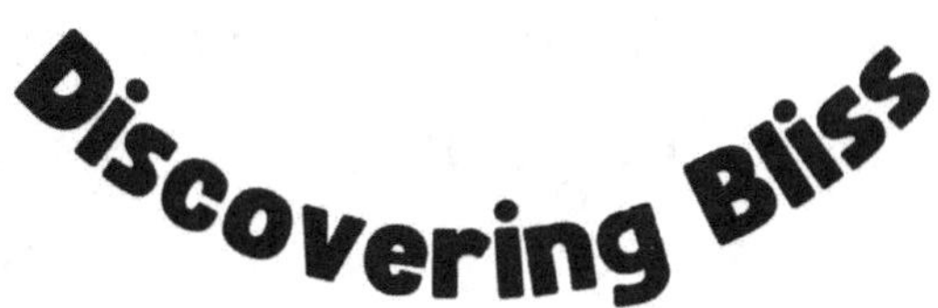

Unveiling the Secrets of What Makes You Happy

Euphoria Mitchell

Copyright © 2023 Euphoria
Mitchell

Euphoria Mitchell

START YOUR DAY WITH HAPPINESS

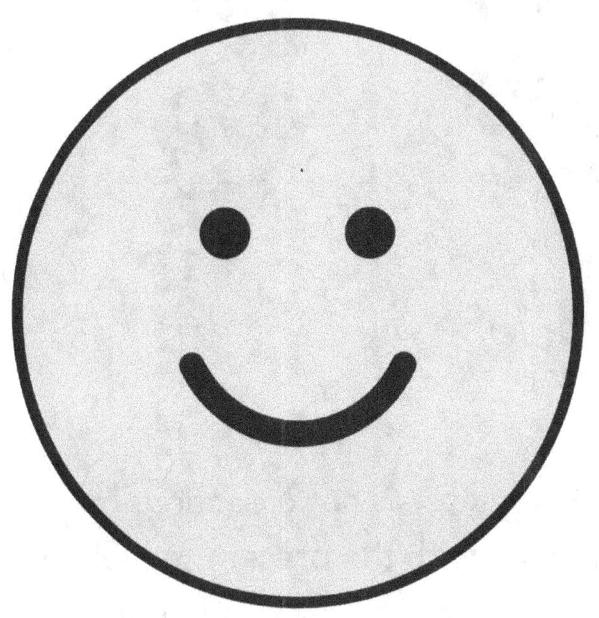

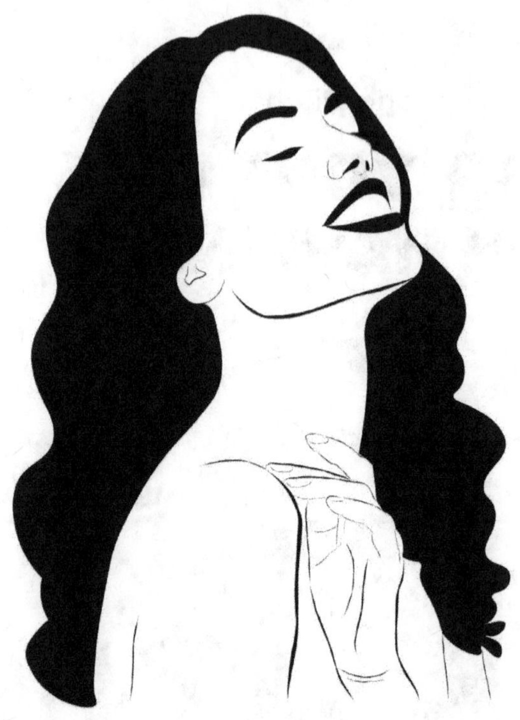

"Happiness is not a destination; it's a dance with the present, a melody of gratitude, and a celebration of the small, beautiful moments that weave the tapestry of our lives." - Euphoria Mitchell

Introducing Euphoria Mitchell, a seasoned happiness therapist with a profound understanding of the intricate nuances that lead fulfilled and joyous life. With a background in psychology and extensive experience in the field, Euphoria has dedicated her career to helping individuals navigate the complexities of their emotional well-being.
Drawing inspiration from her own journey and a genuine passion for uplifting others, Euphoria has become a beacon of positivity in the world of mental health. Her therapeutic approach is marked by a blend of empathy, practical wisdom, and evidence-based techniques, providing her clients with the tools to cultivate happiness from within.
Euphoria Mitchell is not just an author; she is a compassionate guide who has touched the lives of many through her counseling sessions, workshops, and public speaking engagements. Her writing reflects a deep commitment to unraveling the secrets of happiness, offering readers insightful perspectives, actionable advice, and a roadmap to rediscovering joy in their own lives.

HAPPINESS IS FREE

TABLE OF CONTENTS......................

EXCERPT OF THE BOOK..................

The Essence of Happiness:

Explore the fundamental nature of happiness and its significance in our lives. Delve into the science and philosophy behind what it means to be truly happy.

Self-Discovery:

Embark on a self-discovery voyage to understand your own desires, passions, and values. Through introspective exercises and thought-provoking questions, readers will uncover what resonates with their authentic selves.

Mindfulness and Gratitude:

Dive into the practices of mindfulness and gratitude, discovering how they can be powerful tools in cultivating happiness. Learn to appreciate the present moment and find joy in the simple pleasures of life.

Building Meaningful Connections:

Explore the role of relationships in our happiness. From nurturing existing connections to forming new ones, this section provides insights into fostering fulfilling relationships that contribute to overall well-being.

Pursuing Passion and Purpose:

Uncover the connection between passion, purpose, and happiness. Through real-life stories and inspirational examples, readers will be motivated to align their lives with their passions and purpose.

Overcoming Challenges:

Address common obstacles to happiness and learn effective strategies to overcome them. Whether it's stress, fear, or uncertainty, this section offers practical advice on navigating life's challenges.

The Art of Balance:

Understand the importance of balance in various aspects of life, including work, relationships, and personal well-being. Discover how finding equilibrium can contribute to sustained happiness.

Creating Your Happiness Blueprint:

Synthesize the knowledge gained throughout the book to create a personalized happiness blueprint. This actionable plan will guide readers in making intentional choices that align with their newfound understanding of happiness.

Introduction: Unlocking the Doors to Joy

In the pursuit of a meaningful and fulfilling life, there exists a universal quest that transcends time, culture, and individual differences—an unwavering desire for happiness. It is a pursuit that weaves through the tapestry of our existence, coloring the moments of our journey with its radiant hues. Yet, despite its omnipresence, happiness remains an enigma—a concept that is both deeply personal and universally sought after.

"Discovering Bliss" invites you to embark on a transformative exploration, a journey that goes beyond the surface of everyday smiles and ephemeral joys. This is not merely a guide; it is an immersive experience designed to unravel the layers of happiness, revealing the essence that resides within.

The Essence of Happiness: Unveiling the Mystery

In the opening chapter, we dive headfirst into the heart of the matter—what truly constitutes the essence of happiness. We navigate the intricate web of definitions, perspectives, and ideologies surrounding this elusive emotion, seeking to understand its profound significance in our lives.

As we embark on this odyssey, we will:

Defy Definitions:

> Question traditional definitions of happiness and invite you to construct your own understanding. Is it a fleeting emotion, a sustained state of being, or perhaps a delicate dance between the two?

Navigate the Neurological Landscape:

Peer into the intricate realm of neuroscience, exploring the science behind happiness. Discover how our brains, neurotransmitters, and psychological processes orchestrate the symphony of emotions that contribute to our sense of well-being.

Draw Wisdom from the Ages:

Time-travel through philosophical epochs, from ancient wisdom to contemporary thought. Absorb insights from Aristotle's eudaimonia and modern philosophical perspectives, each shedding light on the age-old question of what it means to live a fulfilling life.

Embark on a Cultural Odyssey:

Take a global expedition to understand happiness across cultures. Through this exploration, we aim to broaden perspectives, appreciating the diverse ways in which societies prioritize and pursue happiness.

Weigh Pleasure Against Meaning:

Engage in the debate between the pursuit of pleasure and the quest for meaning. Contemplate the delicate balance between momentary gratification and the sustained fulfillment derived from a life imbued with purpose.

Navigate the Paradox of Choice:

Confront the paradox of choice and its implications on happiness. Learn to discern amidst the abundance, unraveling the complexities that may hinder the pursuit of a simpler, more joyous life.

Embark on Your Personal Odyssey

As we navigate these themes, "Discovering Bliss" lays the groundwork for a personal odyssey—an expedition to uncover the unique elements that compose your happiness. Through introspective exercises, cultural exploration, and philosophical contemplation, you will be equipped with the tools to embark on a self-discovery journey.

This book is not just a guide; it is a companion on your quest for joy. So, let the journey begin—unlock the doors to joy and discover the essence of happiness that resides within you.

Let's dive into the breakdown of Chapter 1, titled "The Essence of Happiness."

1. Defining Happiness:

Objective: Challenge traditional definitions of happiness and encourage readers to construct their own understanding.

Approach: The chapter opens by prompting readers to question common definitions of happiness. Through thought-provoking exercises, readers reflect on what happiness means to them personally. Is it a fleeting emotion, a sustained state of being, or a combination of both?

2. The Science of Happiness:

Objective: Explore the scientific aspects of happiness, examining the role of neuroscience and psychology.

Approach: Delve into the fascinating world of brain chemistry and psychology to understand how positive emotions are generated. Real-life examples and studies are used to illustrate the impact of happiness on physical and mental well-being.

3. Philosophical Insights:

Objective: Draw wisdom from various philosophical perspectives throughout history to enrich the understanding of happiness.

Approach: Take a journey through time, exploring ancient and contemporary philosophical perspectives on happiness. Concepts such as Aristotle's eudaimonia are introduced, providing readers with diverse philosophical insights into the nature of a fulfilling life.

4. Happiness Across Cultures:

Objective: Investigate how different cultures perceive and pursue happiness.

Approach: Through a global exploration, readers gain insights into the cultural variations in the pursuit of happiness. By understanding how societies prioritize and define happiness, readers are encouraged to broaden their perspectives and appreciate the diversity of human experiences.

5. The Pursuit of Pleasure vs. Meaning:

Objective: Engage in the debate between seeking pleasure and pursuing a meaningful life for sustained happiness.

Approach: Readers are prompted to contemplate the balance between momentary pleasures and the enduring fulfillment derived from a purpose-driven life. Through real-world examples and philosophical discussions, the chapter encourages thoughtful consideration of the paths to lasting happiness.

6. The Paradox of Choice:

Objective: Explore how an abundance of choices can impact happiness.

Approach: The chapter addresses the paradox of choice, examining how having too many options can lead to decision fatigue and dissatisfaction. Readers learn strategies to simplify their lives, making choices that align with their values and contribute to overall well-being.

Exercises and Reflections:

Objective: Engage readers in practical exercises and reflections to apply the chapter's concepts to their lives.

Approach: Throughout the chapter, readers encounter exercises and reflective prompts. These activities encourage personal introspection, allowing readers to connect the theoretical concepts discussed with their own experiences and perceptions of happiness.

By the end of Chapter 1, readers have navigated a diverse landscape of ideas and perspectives, laying the groundwork for their personal journey of self-discovery. The chapter sets the stage for the remainder of the book, where readers will build on this foundation to uncover the unique elements that contribute to their own happiness.

Euphoria Mitchell

START YOUR DAY WITH HAPPINESS

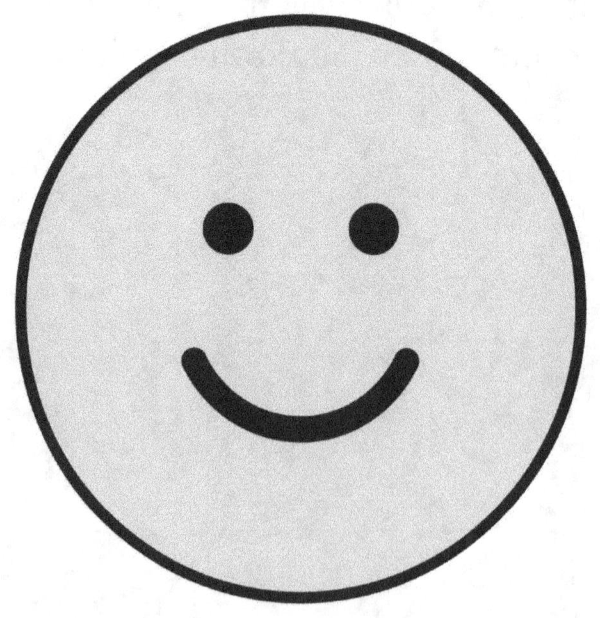

Chapter 2: The Science of Happiness

In the tapestry of human emotion, happiness stands as a beacon—a complex interplay of biology and psychology that shapes our well-being. In this chapter, we embark on a fascinating exploration of the scientific dimensions that underpin the elusive emotion we all seek—happiness.

Diving into Brain Chemistry

As we peel back the layers of understanding, our journey commences in the intricate world of neuroscience. The brain, that enigmatic organ, orchestrates the symphony of emotions. We acquaint ourselves with neurotransmitters—those messengers of joy such as dopamine and serotonin. Through their intricate dance, they weave the fabric of our emotional experiences.

Realizing the Chemistry of Joy:
We delve into the chemical ballet within our brains, understanding how specific neurotransmitters influence our emotional states. Real-life examples illuminate how activities and experiences trigger the release of these chemicals, offering insights into the ways we can intentionally cultivate happiness.

Understanding Psychological Processes

Beyond the realm of neurotransmitters lies the vast landscape of psychology. Positive psychology, a guiding light in this exploration, reveals the profound impact of mindset and thought patterns on our well-being. As we navigate through this psychological terrain, readers gain tools to shape their mental landscapes, fostering a positive and resilient mindset.

Exploring the Mind's Role:
Through engaging narratives and practical

exercises, we unravel the intricate relationship between thoughts and emotions. Readers are invited to reflect on their own cognitive patterns, empowering them to reshape their mental narratives for a happier existence.

Real-Life Examples: Bridging Science and Experience

To bridge the gap between theory and practice, we turn our gaze to real-life examples. Case studies unfold, revealing the transformative power of understanding the science of happiness. These stories serve as beacons, guiding readers toward practical applications of this knowledge in their own lives.

Applying Science to Everyday Life:
Readers are encouraged to draw inspiration from these examples, contemplating how small shifts in behavior and mindset can yield profound effects on their overall happiness. This chapter serves not only as

an exploration of theory but as a guide to actionable steps grounded in scientific understanding.

Impact on Physical and Mental Well-being

Our journey through the science of happiness extends beyond the confines of the mind. We explore the symbiotic relationship between happiness and health—both mental and physical. Scientific studies illuminate the far-reaching benefits of positive emotions, underscoring the importance of a holistic approach to well-being.

Creating a Holistic Perspective:
Readers gain insights into how their emotional well-being influences their physical health and vice versa. Practical strategies for integrating this holistic perspective into daily life are woven into the narrative, empowering readers to embrace a

more comprehensive approach to their happiness journey.

Practical Applications: Nurturing Happiness in Daily Life

Armed with newfound knowledge, we transition from theory to practice. This section is not a mere intellectual exercise but a call to action. Practical applications of the science of happiness are unveiled—mindfulness practices, positive habit cultivation, and the fostering of a growth mindset become tools for readers to wield in their pursuit of joy.

Empowering Choices:
Readers are invited to reflect on how these practical applications align with their unique circumstances. Each strategy becomes a brushstroke in the canvas of their lives, allowing them to actively participate in the creation of their own happiness narrative.

This chapter serves as a bridge between the theoretical and the practical, grounding readers in the scientific underpinnings of happiness while providing actionable steps for its cultivation. The narrative flows seamlessly, inviting readers to not only understand the science of happiness but to actively engage with it in their daily lives.

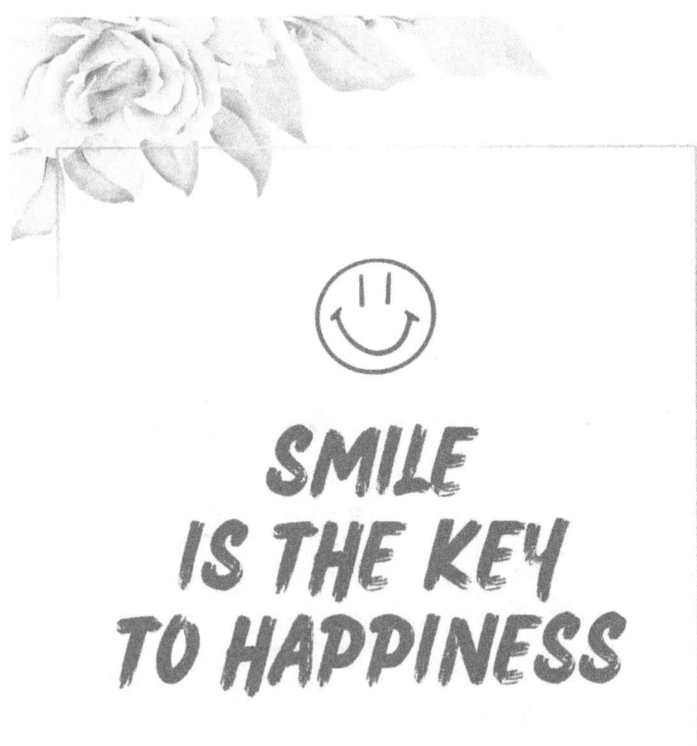

EUPHORIA MITCHELL

3. Philosophical Insights:

Draw wisdom from various philosophical perspectives throughout history to enrich the understanding of happiness.

Approach:

Embarking on a Journey Through Time

In this chapter, we embark on a philosophical odyssey—a timeless exploration of the profound insights and timeless wisdom offered by thinkers across the ages. As we traverse the annals of philosophy, we seek to deepen our understanding of happiness and glean valuable lessons from the enduring wisdom of philosophers.

Ancient Wisdom: Aristotle's Eudaimonia

Our journey begins with Aristotle, the ancient Greek philosopher whose musings on eudaimonia, or "flourishing," remain remarkably relevant. Through the lens of Aristotle's teachings, we delve into the concept of a life well-lived—one characterized by the pursuit of virtue, personal growth, and the realization of one's true potential.

Practical Application:
Readers are invited to reflect on how the principles of eudaimonia align with their own values and aspirations. Through practical exercises, they can begin to envision a life infused with purpose and meaning.

Eastern Philosophy: Embracing Zen and Balance

The philosophical exploration extends beyond the Western tradition to embrace the wisdom of Eastern philosophy. Zen teachings guide us towards the importance of balance, mindfulness, and living in the present moment. We unravel the art of finding contentment in simplicity and serenity.

Applying Zen Wisdom:
Practical applications rooted in Zen philosophy are introduced. Readers are encouraged to integrate principles of balance and mindfulness into their daily routines, fostering a sense of tranquility and harmony.

Existentialism: Finding Meaning in the Absurd

In the existentialist realm, we confront the challenges posed by the absurdity of existence. Thinkers like Jean-Paul Sartre and Albert Camus prompt us to grapple with the inherent meaninglessness of life and find purpose in the face of this existential void.

Navigating Existential Questions:
Through philosophical inquiries, readers are prompted to confront existential questions and consider how they personally derive meaning in the midst of life's uncertainties. The chapter serves as a catalyst for readers to forge their own paths to meaning and purpose.

Modern Perspectives: Positive Psychology and Beyond

Our journey concludes with a glance at modern perspectives, particularly the emergence of positive psychology. We explore how contemporary thinkers have built upon ancient wisdom, blending traditional philosophy with empirical research to create a holistic understanding of happiness.

Synthesizing Ancient and Modern Wisdom:
Readers are encouraged to synthesize insights from both ancient and modern philosophies, creating a rich tapestry of

understanding. The chapter sets the stage for a personalized integration of philosophical principles into the reader's own pursuit of happiness.

In this chapter, readers not only gain intellectual insights into different philosophical traditions but are also provided with practical applications and reflections that bridge the gap between ancient wisdom and the complexities of modern life. The philosophical journey becomes a guide, offering diverse perspectives for readers to consider on their quest for happiness.

HAPPINESS IS FREE

4. Happiness Across Cultures:

Investigate how different cultures perceive and pursue happiness.

Approach:

Cultural Explorations:

In this chapter, we embark on a cultural odyssey, exploring how diverse societies around the world conceptualize and seek happiness. By understanding the cultural variations in the pursuit of joy, readers gain a broader perspective on the universal quest for well-being.

Eastern Philosophies: Harmony and Inner Peace

Our journey commences with a look at Eastern cultures, where philosophies such as Confucianism and Taoism emphasize harmony, balance, and inner peace. Through cultural narratives and traditions, readers gain insights into how these principles shape the pursuit of happiness in Eastern societies.

Applying Eastern Wisdom:
Practical applications draw from Eastern philosophies, encouraging readers to incorporate principles of harmony and balance into their lives. The chapter serves as a bridge between cultural insights and actionable steps for readers seeking a more balanced and harmonious existence.

Nordic Happiness: Hygge and Social Connection

The exploration extends to Nordic cultures, where concepts like hygge emphasize coziness, connection, and a sense of community. Through real-life examples, readers discover how social bonds and embracing simple pleasures contribute to the well-being of individuals in Nordic societies.

Cultivating Hygge in Daily Life:
Readers are invited to reflect on how they can infuse elements of hygge into their own lives. This section serves as a guide for creating environments and fostering connections that contribute to a warm and contented existence.

Bhutan's Gross National Happiness: A Holistic Approach

The chapter takes a detour to Bhutan, a country that measures its success through Gross National Happiness (GNH). By examining Bhutan's unique approach, readers gain insights into a holistic perspective that includes not only economic factors but also spiritual, cultural, and environmental dimensions.

Reflecting on Personal Values:
Through guided reflections, readers evaluate the holistic dimensions of their own lives. What elements contribute to their overall happiness, and how can they align their

pursuits with a more comprehensive understanding of well-being?

Individualism vs. Collectivism: Cultural Influences

The exploration delves into the cultural dichotomy of individualism and collectivism. By comparing cultures that emphasize individual achievement with those that prioritize communal well-being, readers gain an understanding of how cultural values shape the pursuit and perception of happiness.

Navigating Cultural Influences:
Practical exercises encourage readers to navigate their own cultural influences. How do societal expectations and cultural values impact their personal definitions of happiness, and how can they navigate these influences to create a more authentic and fulfilling life?

Global Insights: A Mosaic of Happiness

The chapter concludes by synthesizing global insights into a mosaic of happiness. By appreciating the diverse ways in which cultures approach well-being, readers are empowered to draw inspiration from different traditions, creating a personalized and culturally informed approach to happiness.

In this chapter, readers embark on a journey around the globe, gaining cultural perspectives that enrich their understanding of happiness. Practical applications and reflections guide readers in integrating these insights into their own pursuit of joy, fostering a more nuanced and culturally aware approach to well-being.

5. The Pursuit of Pleasure vs. Meaning:

Engage in the debate between seeking pleasure and pursuing a meaningful life for sustained happiness.

Approach:

Balancing Pleasure and Meaning:

In this chapter, we confront a pivotal question that echoes through the corridors of philosophy and psychology: Is happiness derived from the pursuit of pleasure, or does a meaningful life hold the key to enduring fulfillment? Our exploration navigates the delicate balance between momentary gratification and the pursuit of profound purpose.

The Pleasure Principle: Hedonism Revisited

Our journey begins by revisiting hedonism, the age-old philosophy that places pleasure at the forefront of the pursuit of happiness. Through historical perspectives and contemporary insights, readers gain an understanding of how the pursuit of pleasure, in its various forms, influences our well-being.

Navigating Pleasure-Seeking Behaviors: Practical reflections prompt readers to evaluate their own tendencies toward seeking pleasure. How do immediate gratifications impact their overall happiness, and what role do these pleasures play in their lives?

The Quest for Meaning: Victor Frankl's Logotherapy

We shift our focus to the profound teachings of Viktor Frankl and logotherapy—a philosophy that places meaning and purpose as central to human existence. Through Frankl's poignant narrative and philosophical insights, readers are prompted to consider how a life infused with meaning contributes to sustained happiness.

Crafting Personal Meaning:

Guided exercises encourage readers to delve into their own sense of purpose. What gives their lives meaning, and how can they align their pursuits with a deeper, more enduring source of happiness?

Striking a Balance: The Psychology of Well-being

The exploration continues by delving into contemporary psychological perspectives that seek a harmonious balance between pleasure and meaning. Positive psychology, in particular, offers insights into how individuals can cultivate both hedonic and eudaimonic well-being for a more holistic sense of happiness.

Integrating Pleasure and Purpose:

Readers are empowered to integrate pleasure and purpose into their lives. Practical strategies guide them in finding a delicate equilibrium, where momentary joys coexist with the pursuit of long-term fulfillment.

The Paradox of Hedonic Adaptation: Navigating Change

Our journey concludes with an exploration of the paradox of hedonic adaptation—the phenomenon wherein the thrill of pleasurable experiences diminishes over time. Readers learn to navigate this paradox, understanding how adaptation influences their pursuit of pleasure and discovering ways to infuse novelty and variety into their lives.

Embracing Change for Lasting Happiness: Reflective exercises guide readers in embracing change as a catalyst for sustained happiness. How can they introduce variety and novelty into their lives to counteract the effects of hedonic adaptation?

Creating a Personal Synthesis: Pleasure and Purpose Unveiled

The chapter concludes by inviting readers to synthesize their insights into a personalized approach to happiness. By striking a balance between the pursuit of pleasure and the cultivation of meaning, readers are empowered to craft a unique and sustainable path to enduring well-being.

In this chapter, readers grapple with fundamental questions about the nature of happiness, exploring the interplay between pleasure and meaning. Through a blend of historical perspectives, psychological insights, and practical exercises, readers emerge equipped to navigate the intricate dance between immediate gratification and the pursuit of lasting fulfillment.

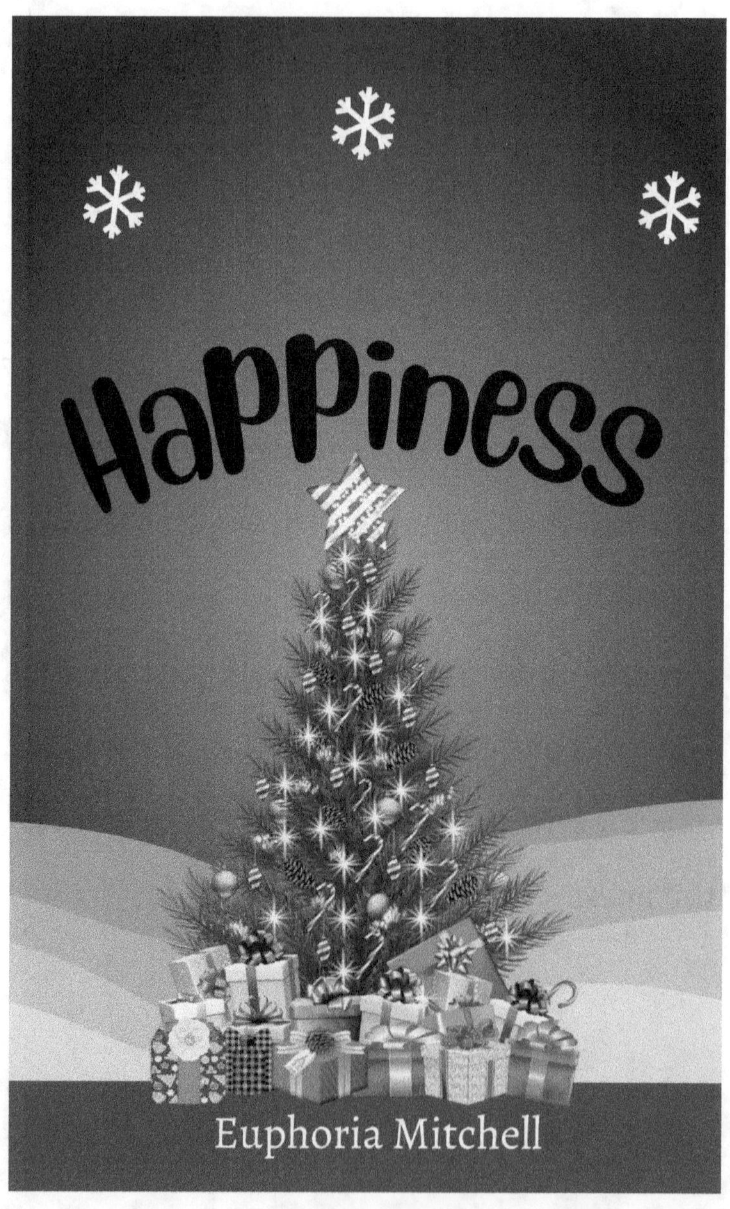
Happiness
Euphoria Mitchell

6. The Paradox of Choice

Explore how an abundance of choices can impact happiness and learn strategies to simplify life for enhanced well-being.

Approach:

Navigating the Sea of Choices:

This chapter delves into the paradox of choice—an exploration of how an abundance of options can affect our ability to make decisions and influence our overall sense of happiness. As we sail through the sea of choices, we seek to understand the complexities that arise when confronted with an overwhelming array of options.

The Burden of Endless Options:

Our journey begins with an examination of the psychological burden that arises when faced with an excess of choices. Drawing on insights from psychology and behavioral economics, readers gain an understanding of decision fatigue and the emotional toll of navigating an infinite sea of options.

Navigating Decision Fatigue:
Practical reflections guide readers in recognizing instances of decision fatigue in their lives. How do the choices they make daily impact their well-being, and how can they mitigate the effects of decision overload?

Simplifying Life: Embracing Minimalism and Essentialism:

In response to the paradox of choice, we explore the principles of minimalism and essentialism. By simplifying life and focusing on what truly matters, readers learn how to declutter their physical and mental spaces, creating room for clarity and contentment.

Practical Steps to Simplify:
Readers are invited to engage in practical

exercises that guide them in simplifying various aspects of their lives. From decluttering physical spaces to streamlining daily routines, the chapter serves as a roadmap to embracing simplicity for enhanced well-being.

Cultivating Gratitude in the Midst of Abundance:

The exploration extends to the concept of gratitude—a powerful antidote to the challenges posed by excessive choices. By fostering an attitude of gratitude, readers learn to appreciate the abundance in their lives without being overwhelmed by it.

Gratitude Practices:
Guided exercises introduce readers to gratitude practices that can be seamlessly integrated into their daily lives. These practices become anchors, grounding individuals in a positive mindset amidst the complexities of choice.

Mindful Decision-Making: Finding Clarity Amidst Complexity:

Mindfulness becomes a guiding principle as we navigate the complexities of decision-making. By cultivating a mindful approach to choices, readers learn to make decisions with greater intentionality, reducing stress and fostering a deeper sense of well-being.

Incorporating Mindfulness:
Practical applications introduce readers to mindfulness techniques that enhance their ability to make conscious and meaningful choices. From mindful breathing to reflective decision-making, readers discover the transformative power of mindfulness.

The Art of Saying "No":

Our journey concludes with an exploration of the liberating art of saying "no." Readers are empowered to set boundaries, prioritize what truly matters, and recognize that opting out of certain choices can be a powerful act of self-care.

Setting Boundaries:
Reflection exercises guide readers in evaluating their own boundaries and exploring instances where saying "no" can contribute to a more intentional and fulfilling life.

In this chapter, readers navigate the intricacies of choice, learning to mitigate decision fatigue, embrace simplicity, and cultivate gratitude. Through practical applications and mindfulness practices, they emerge equipped to navigate the paradox of choice and make decisions that align with their values and contribute to their overall well-being.

7. Embark on Your Personal Odyssey:

Begin a personal journey of self-discovery, using the insights gained to uncover the unique elements that contribute to your happiness.

Approach:

Charting Your Course:

This chapter marks the beginning of a transformative personal odyssey. Armed with the knowledge gained from previous chapters, readers are now invited to embark on a journey of self-discovery—a process that goes beyond theory and invites them to actively shape their own narratives of happiness.

Reflecting on Moments of True Happiness:

Our journey commences with a deep dive into personal experiences. Through reflective exercises, readers are encouraged to explore and identify moments in their lives when they experienced genuine happiness. These reflections serve as beacons, guiding readers towards understanding the unique elements that contribute to their well-being.

Creating a Happiness Journal:

Practical applications guide readers in

creating a happiness journal—a tangible record of moments that evoke joy. This exercise becomes a valuable resource for self-discovery, enabling readers to identify patterns and themes in their sources of happiness.

Exploring Values and Priorities:

The odyssey extends to the exploration of values and priorities. Readers are prompted to examine their core values and assess how well their current life aligns with these foundational principles. By understanding what truly matters, readers gain clarity on the aspects of life that contribute to their overall sense of happiness.

Values Assessment:

Reflective exercises guide readers through a values assessment, providing a framework for aligning their daily choices with their core values. This exploration becomes a compass, directing them towards a life that resonates with authenticity.

Cultivating Flow and Engagement:

The chapter introduces the concept of "flow"—a state of complete immersion and energized focus. Through practical applications, readers discover activities that induce a sense of flow, contributing to a heightened sense of fulfillment and happiness.

Discovering Personal Flow Activities:
Guided exercises lead readers in discovering their own flow-inducing activities. This exploration becomes a dynamic aspect of their happiness journey, fostering a sense of engagement and purpose.

Building Meaningful Connections:

The odyssey takes a relational turn as we explore the role of connections in happiness. By examining the quality of relationships and assessing social connections, readers gain insights into the impact of interpersonal dynamics on their well-being.

Assessing Social Networks:
Practical reflections guide readers in

assessing the quality of their social networks. By nurturing meaningful connections and setting boundaries in toxic relationships, readers actively shape their social landscapes for greater happiness.

Setting Personal Goals for Joy:

Our journey concludes with the setting of personal goals. Readers are encouraged to translate their newfound insights into actionable steps, setting realistic and meaningful goals that align with their values and contribute to their overall happiness.

Goal-Setting for Well-being:

Guided exercises lead readers in setting personal goals that encompass various aspects of their lives. From career aspirations to personal growth objectives, these goals become the milestones of their ongoing happiness journey.

In this chapter, readers transition from theoretical understanding to practical application, embarking on a personal odyssey of self-discovery. The exercises and reflections guide them in uncovering the unique elements that contribute to their happiness, empowering them to actively shape their lives in alignment with their values and aspirations.

8. The Art of Mindfulness:

Explore the transformative power of mindfulness in enhancing well-being and happiness.

Approach:

Cultivating Present-Moment Awareness:

In this chapter, we delve into the art of mindfulness—a practice that has the potential to profoundly impact well-being. By cultivating present-moment awareness, readers discover how mindfulness can serve as a powerful tool in navigating the complexities of life and fostering a deeper sense of happiness.

Understanding Mindfulness:

Our journey begins with an exploration of the fundamental principles of mindfulness. Readers are introduced to the concept of non-judgmental awareness, observing thoughts and sensations without attachment. Through anecdotes and real-life examples, the chapter demystifies mindfulness and its relevance to happiness.

Mindfulness in Everyday Life:
Practical applications guide readers in incorporating mindfulness into their daily routines. From mindful breathing exercises to simple techniques for staying present, readers are equipped with tools to enhance their awareness in the midst of life's activities.

Mindful Living: Bringing Awareness to Daily Activities:

The exploration extends to the practice of mindful living—a conscious approach to daily activities. Readers learn to infuse ordinary moments with mindfulness, transforming routine actions into opportunities for presence and appreciation.

Mindful Eating, Walking, and Listening:
Guided exercises lead readers in applying mindfulness to activities such as eating, walking, and listening. By savoring the richness of each moment, readers cultivate a heightened sense of awareness and connection to their surroundings.

Mindfulness for Stress Reduction:

The chapter addresses the role of mindfulness in stress reduction. Readers gain insights into how mindful practices can mitigate the impact of stress on mental and physical well-being. Through mindfulness-based stress reduction techniques, readers build resilience and a more adaptive response to life's challenges.

Stress-Reduction Techniques:
Practical exercises guide readers in incorporating mindfulness into

stress-inducing situations. From mindful breathing to body scan meditation, readers develop a repertoire of techniques for navigating stress with grace and resilience.

Mindfulness and Emotional Well-being:

Our journey takes a deeper dive into the connection between mindfulness and emotional well-being. Readers explore how cultivating mindfulness can enhance emotional intelligence, allowing for a more balanced and intentional response to emotions.

Cultivating Emotional Awareness:
Guided reflections lead readers in cultivating emotional awareness through mindfulness. By observing and understanding their emotional landscape, readers develop a greater capacity for emotional regulation and resilience.

Mindfulness for Enhanced Relationships:

The exploration concludes with the impact of mindfulness on relationships. By bringing mindful awareness to interpersonal interactions, readers foster deeper connections and communication. The chapter explores how mindfulness contributes to empathy, compassion, and overall relational well-being.

Mindful Communication:
Practical applications guide readers in incorporating mindful communication into their relationships. From active listening to compassionate responses, readers enhance the quality of their connections with others.

In this chapter, readers immerse themselves in the transformative practice of mindfulness, discovering its relevance to happiness, stress reduction, emotional well-being, and interpersonal relationships.

Practical exercises empower readers to integrate mindfulness into various aspects of their lives, fostering a profound sense of awareness and presence.

9. Gratitude Unveiled:

Explore the transformative power of gratitude in cultivating a positive mindset and enhancing overall well-being.

Approach:

Unlocking the Gift of Gratitude:

This chapter delves into the profound practice of gratitude—a timeless principle that has the potential to shift perspectives and elevate the human experience. Readers embark on a journey to unlock the gift of gratitude and discover its transformative impact on well-being.

Understanding the Essence of Gratitude:

Our exploration begins with a deep dive into the essence of gratitude. Readers uncover the psychological and emotional dimensions of gratitude, understanding how this practice extends beyond polite gestures to become a cornerstone of a positive and fulfilling life.

Gratitude as a Mindset:
Practical reflections guide readers in adopting a mindset of gratitude. By recognizing and appreciating the positive aspects of their lives, readers lay the foundation for a more optimistic and joy-filled existence.

Gratitude Practices: From Journaling to Rituals:

The chapter introduces various gratitude practices that readers can incorporate into their daily lives. From gratitude journaling to creating gratitude rituals, readers discover diverse ways to express and cultivate gratitude, enhancing their overall sense of appreciation.

Creating a Gratitude Journal:
Guided exercises lead readers in

establishing their own gratitude journal. This personalized practice becomes a sacred space for acknowledging and celebrating the abundance in their lives, fostering a continuous awareness of gratitude.

Gratitude and Resilience:

The exploration extends to the role of gratitude in building resilience. By reframing challenges through a lens of gratitude, readers learn to navigate adversity with a greater sense of perspective and fortitude.

Cultivating Resilience Through Gratitude: Practical applications guide readers in applying gratitude to challenging situations. By acknowledging lessons, finding silver linings, and expressing gratitude in the face of adversity, readers enhance their capacity for resilience.

Gratitude in Relationships: Fostering Connection:

Our journey takes a relational turn as we explore the impact of gratitude on interpersonal connections. Readers discover how expressing gratitude can strengthen relationships, foster goodwill, and contribute to a positive and supportive social environment.

Expressing Gratitude to Others:
Guided reflections lead readers in expressing gratitude to those around them. From friends and family to colleagues and acquaintances, readers learn to articulate and share their appreciation, deepening the bonds of connection.

Gratitude and Self-Reflection:

The chapter concludes with an exploration of gratitude as a tool for self-reflection. By appreciating personal growth and achievements, readers cultivate a positive self-image and a sense of fulfillment.

Gratitude for Personal Growth:
Practical exercises guide readers in practicing self-reflective gratitude. By acknowledging and celebrating their own progress, readers foster a positive self-narrative and a deeper connection to their own journeys.

In this chapter, readers unravel the transformative power of gratitude—a practice that extends beyond mere acknowledgment to become a mindset and a way of life. Practical applications and reflective exercises empower readers to integrate gratitude into various facets of their lives, fostering positivity, resilience, and deeper connections with others.

CONTROL YOURSELF TO BE HAPPY

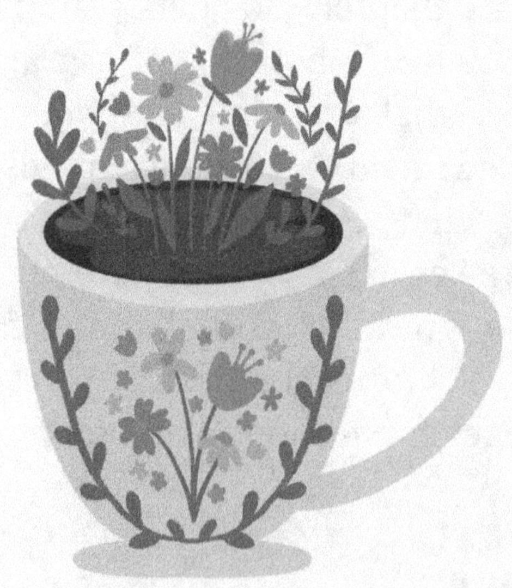

MAURELL MAVIN

10. The Impact of Positive Habits:

Explore the science of habit formation and its role in cultivating a positive and fulfilling life.

Approach:

The Power of Habits: A Foundation for Well-being:

In this chapter, we delve into the science and psychology of habits—a powerful force that shapes our daily lives. Readers explore the impact of habits on well-being and happiness, learning how intentional habit formation can be a catalyst for positive change.

Understanding Habit Loops:

Our journey begins with an exploration of habit loops, comprising cues, routines, and rewards. Readers gain insights into the neurological and psychological mechanisms that drive habit formation, empowering them to understand and shape their own behavior.

Identifying Habit Loops:
Practical exercises guide readers in identifying existing habit loops in their lives. By recognizing cues, routines, and rewards, readers gain a deeper understanding of the automatic patterns that influence their daily actions.

Positive Habit Formation: A Blueprint for Change:

The chapter introduces the concept of positive habit formation—a deliberate and intentional process of cultivating habits that contribute to well-being. Readers explore the blueprint for creating positive habits, understanding the key elements that lead to successful habit formation.

Creating a Habit Blueprint:
Guided reflections lead readers in creating their own habit blueprints. From setting clear intentions to incorporating gradual changes, readers develop a roadmap for cultivating positive habits aligned with their goals and values.

Habits for Physical Well-being:

Our exploration extends to the impact of habits on physical well-being. Readers discover how small, consistent changes in daily routines can lead to significant improvements in health, energy levels, and overall vitality.

Incorporating Healthy Habits:
Practical applications guide readers in incorporating healthy habits into their daily lives. From mindful eating to regular physical activity, readers discover how intentional habits contribute to their physical well-being.

Habits for Emotional Resilience:

The chapter addresses the role of habits in emotional resilience. Readers explore how cultivating habits related to self-care, mindfulness, and stress management can enhance their capacity to navigate life's emotional challenges.

Cultivating Emotional Well-being Habits:
Guided exercises lead readers in cultivating habits that contribute to emotional well-being. By integrating practices like gratitude, mindfulness, and self-reflection, readers enhance their emotional resilience and overall happiness.

Social Habits: Nurturing Positive Connections:

Our journey takes a relational turn as we explore the impact of social habits on happiness. Readers learn how intentional habits in interpersonal interactions can strengthen relationships, foster a positive social environment, and contribute to a sense of community.

Nurturing Positive Social Habits:
Practical applications guide readers in nurturing positive social habits. From acts of kindness to intentional communication, readers discover how small gestures can create a ripple effect of positivity in their social circles.

Reflecting on Habit Evolution:

The chapter concludes with a reflection on the evolution of habits. Readers are encouraged to assess and adapt their habits over time, recognizing that personal growth and changing circumstances warrant ongoing adjustments to support their well-being.

Adapting and Evolving Habits:
Guided reflections lead readers in evaluating the effectiveness of their habits and making intentional adjustments. By embracing a

growth mindset, readers cultivate habits that evolve with their changing needs and aspirations.

In this chapter, readers gain a comprehensive understanding of the impact of habits on well-being and happiness. Practical applications and reflective exercises empower readers to intentionally cultivate positive habits in various aspects of their lives, creating a foundation for a positive and fulfilling existence.

11. The Role of Resilience: Building Inner Strength:

Explore the concept of resilience and provide practical strategies for building inner strength in the face of life's challenges.

Approach:

Understanding Resilience: A Beacon in Adversity:

In this chapter, we delve into the concept of resilience—a quality that empowers individuals to bounce back and thrive in the face of adversity. Readers explore the psychological and emotional dimensions of resilience, understanding how it can be cultivated to navigate life's challenges with grace.

The Components of Resilience:

Our journey begins with an exploration of the components that contribute to resilience. Readers gain insights into factors such as adaptability, optimism, social support, and self-regulation that form the foundation of resilience.

Reflecting on Personal Resilience:
Practical exercises guide readers in reflecting on their own resilience. By identifying strengths and areas for growth, readers gain a deeper understanding of their capacity to navigate life's ups and downs.

Cultivating a Growth Mindset: The Foundation of Resilience:

The chapter introduces the concept of a growth mindset—a foundational element of resilience. Readers explore how adopting a mindset that views challenges as opportunities for growth enhances their ability to bounce back from setbacks.

Fostering a Growth Mindset:
Guided reflections lead readers in fostering a growth mindset. By reframing challenges,

embracing learning opportunities, and cultivating a belief in their own capacity to grow, readers build a solid foundation for resilience.

Adapting to Change: The Resilience of Flexibility:

Our exploration extends to the resilience of flexibility—navigating change with adaptability and openness. Readers learn how the ability to adjust to new circumstances contributes to resilience and fosters a sense of control in the face of uncertainty.

Embracing Adaptive Strategies:
Practical applications guide readers in embracing adaptive strategies. From cultivating flexibility in thinking to adjusting goals and expectations, readers develop tools for navigating change with resilience.

Building Social Support Networks: The Resilience of Connection:

The chapter addresses the crucial role of social support in resilience. Readers explore how nurturing positive relationships and seeking support from others contribute to their ability to face challenges with resilience.

Strengthening Social Connections:
Guided exercises lead readers in strengthening their social support networks. By fostering positive connections and communicating effectively with others, readers enhance their resilience through the power of relationships.

Mindfulness and Resilience: A Unified Approach:

Our journey takes a mindful turn as we explore the intersection of mindfulness and resilience. Readers discover how cultivating present-moment awareness and mindfulness practices can fortify their inner strength in the face of adversity.

Integrating Mindfulness for Resilience:
Practical applications guide readers in integrating mindfulness practices into their resilience-building toolkit. From mindful breathing to acceptance of difficult emotions, readers develop a holistic approach to inner strength.

Coping Strategies for Emotional Resilience:

The chapter addresses coping strategies for emotional resilience. Readers explore techniques for managing stress, regulating emotions, and cultivating a positive outlook, equipping them with tools to navigate emotional challenges with resilience.

Practical Coping Exercises:
Guided exercises lead readers in practicing coping strategies for emotional resilience. From stress-reducing activities to positive

affirmations, readers develop a personalized toolkit for emotional well-being.

Reflecting on Personal Resilience Stories:

The chapter concludes with an invitation for readers to reflect on personal stories of resilience. By recalling and celebrating instances of overcoming challenges, readers reinforce their belief in their own resilience and draw inspiration for future endeavors.

Creating a Resilience Journal:
Guided reflections lead readers in creating a resilience journal—a tangible record of their resilience stories. This exercise becomes a source of inspiration and a reminder of their inner strength.

In this chapter, readers embark on a journey to understand and cultivate resilience—a quality that empowers individuals to face life's challenges with strength and grace.

Practical applications and reflective exercises guide readers in building inner strength and developing resilience as a cornerstone of their well-being.

12. The Art of Self-Compassion: Nurturing the Inner Self:

Explore the concept of self-compassion and provide practical strategies for cultivating kindness and understanding towards oneself.

Approach:

Embracing Self-Compassion: A Path to Inner Healing:

In this chapter, we delve into the art of self-compassion—a transformative practice that involves treating oneself with kindness and understanding, especially in moments of difficulty. Readers explore the emotional and psychological dimensions of self-compassion and its profound impact on well-being.

Understanding the Components of Self-Compassion:

Our journey begins with an exploration of the components that make up self-compassion, as defined by psychologist Kristin Neff. Readers gain insights into self-kindness, common humanity, and mindfulness—the pillars that form the foundation of a compassionate relationship with oneself.

Reflecting on Self-Compassion:
Practical exercises guide readers in reflecting on their own relationship with self-compassion. By identifying areas of strength and areas for growth, readers set the stage for cultivating a more compassionate inner dialogue.

Practicing Self-Kindness: The Heart of Self-Compassion:

The chapter introduces the practice of self-kindness—the act of treating oneself with warmth and understanding. Readers explore how self-kindness serves as a source of comfort and support, particularly during challenging times.

Cultivating Self-Kindness:
Guided reflections lead readers in cultivating self-kindness through practical exercises. From positive affirmations to acts of self-care, readers develop personalized strategies for integrating kindness into their daily lives.

Common Humanity: Connecting Through Shared Experiences:

Our exploration extends to the concept of common humanity—a recognition that challenges and difficulties are part of the shared human experience. Readers discover how acknowledging common humanity fosters a sense of connection and reduces feelings of isolation.

Affirming Common Humanity:
Practical applications guide readers in affirming their common humanity with others. Through exercises that emphasize shared experiences and interconnectedness, readers cultivate a sense of belonging and understanding.

Mindfulness and Self-Compassion: A Unified Presence:

The chapter addresses the intersection of mindfulness and self-compassion. Readers explore how mindfulness practices enhance the ability to approach one's experiences with an open and non-judgmental attitude, fostering self-compassion.

Integrating Mindfulness into Self-Compassion:
Guided exercises lead readers in integrating mindfulness practices into their self-compassion journey. From mindful self-compassion meditations to present-moment awareness, readers

develop a unified approach to nurturing the inner self.

Overcoming Self-Criticism: The Compassionate Response:

Our journey takes on the challenge of overcoming self-criticism—a common barrier to self-compassion. Readers explore strategies for responding to self-critical thoughts with compassion and understanding, promoting a more positive and supportive inner dialogue.

Responding to Self-Criticism:
Practical applications guide readers in responding to self-critical thoughts with compassion. Through cognitive restructuring and self-compassionate language, readers shift the narrative towards a more supportive and nurturing perspective.

Self-Compassion in Action: Navigating Difficult Emotions:

The chapter addresses the application of self-compassion in navigating difficult emotions. Readers explore how self-compassion serves as a resource for managing emotional challenges, allowing for greater resilience and well-being.

Applying Self-Compassion to Difficult Emotions:
Guided exercises lead readers in applying self-compassion to specific difficult emotions. From moments of sadness to experiences of failure, readers cultivate a compassionate response that promotes emotional well-being.

Cultivating a Self-Compassionate Lifestyle:

The chapter concludes with an exploration of cultivating a self-compassionate lifestyle. Readers discover how integrating self-compassion into various aspects of their lives creates a foundation for enhanced well-being and a more positive relationship with themselves.

Creating a Self-Compassionate Action Plan:
Guided reflections lead readers in creating a self-compassionate action plan. By identifying specific areas for improvement and setting realistic goals, readers embark on a journey towards a more compassionate and nurturing lifestyle.

In this chapter, readers explore the transformative practice of self-compassion—a journey of treating oneself with kindness and understanding. Practical applications and reflective exercises guide readers in cultivating self-kindness, acknowledging common humanity, and integrating mindfulness into their daily lives, fostering a more compassionate relationship with the inner self.

13. The Art of Gracious Living: Cultivating a Positive Lifestyle:

Explore the components of a positive lifestyle and provide practical strategies for cultivating gratitude, joy, and meaning in daily living.

Approach:

Gracious Living: Crafting a Positive Lifestyle:

In this chapter, we embark on a journey to explore the art of gracious living—a deliberate and intentional approach to crafting a positive and meaningful lifestyle. Readers discover how small, intentional choices can contribute to a life rich in gratitude, joy, and purpose.

Cultivating Gratitude in Daily Life:

Our journey begins with the exploration of gratitude as a cornerstone of gracious living.

Readers learn how to infuse daily routines with gratitude practices, creating a positive mindset and an appreciation for the richness of life.

Daily Gratitude Rituals:
Practical applications guide readers in incorporating gratitude into their daily lives. From morning gratitude reflections to evening gratitude journals, readers develop rituals that foster a continuous awareness of the blessings in their lives.

Finding Joy in Simple Pleasures: The Power of Delight:

The chapter introduces the concept of finding joy in simple pleasures—a practice that emphasizes the importance of savoring and appreciating the small, everyday moments that bring delight.

Savoring Simple Pleasures:
Guided reflections lead readers in savoring simple pleasures. From mindful moments to

intentional enjoyment of activities, readers cultivate a sense of joy that permeates their daily lives.

Mindful Living: Bringing Presence to Daily Activities:

Our exploration extends to mindful living—a practice that involves bringing present-moment awareness to daily activities. Readers discover how mindfulness enhances the quality of experiences, fostering a deeper connection to the unfolding moments of life.

Incorporating Mindfulness into Daily Activities:
Practical applications guide readers in incorporating mindfulness into various aspects of their daily lives. From mindful eating to mindful communication, readers develop a heightened sense of presence and engagement.

Creating Meaningful Rituals: Enhancing Daily Life with Purpose:

The chapter addresses the importance of creating meaningful rituals—a practice that involves infusing daily routines with intentionality and purpose. Readers explore how rituals contribute to a sense of continuity, meaning, and connection.

Designing Personal Rituals:
Guided exercises lead readers in designing their own meaningful rituals. From morning rituals that set a positive tone to evening rituals that promote reflection and gratitude, readers craft personalized routines that align with their values.

Positive Habits for Health and Well-being:

Our journey takes a holistic turn as we explore positive habits that contribute to health and well-being. Readers discover how intentional choices related to nutrition, exercise, and sleep create a foundation for physical vitality and overall wellness.

Cultivating Positive Health Habits:
Practical applications guide readers in cultivating positive health habits. From mindful eating practices to regular physical activity, readers develop a holistic approach to well-being that supports a positive lifestyle.

Nurturing Positive Relationships: The Heart of Gracious Living:

The chapter addresses the pivotal role of positive relationships in gracious living. Readers explore how intentional efforts to nurture and strengthen relationships contribute to a positive and supportive social environment.

Nurturing Relationships:
Guided reflections lead readers in nurturing positive relationships. From expressing gratitude to active listening, readers

cultivate habits that enhance the quality of their connections with others.

Reflecting on a Gracious Lifestyle: Crafting Your Narrative:

The chapter concludes with an invitation for readers to reflect on their gracious lifestyle. Readers are encouraged to craft their own narratives of gracious living, celebrating the positive choices and intentional practices that contribute to their overall well-being.

Creating a Gracious Living Journal:
Guided reflections lead readers in creating a gracious living journal—a tangible record of their positive choices and lifestyle practices. This exercise becomes a source of inspiration and a reminder of the intentional steps taken toward a more fulfilling and meaningful life.

In this chapter, readers explore the art of gracious living—a deliberate and intentional approach to crafting a positive and meaningful lifestyle. Practical applications and reflective exercises guide readers in cultivating gratitude, joy, and purpose in daily living, creating a foundation for a life rich in meaning and well-being.

14. The Journey Within: Connecting with Your Authentic Self:

Explore the concept of authenticity and provide practical strategies for connecting with one's true self in the journey toward happiness.

Approach:

Authentic Living: Embracing Your True Self:

In this chapter, we embark on a journey to explore the concept of authenticity—a practice that involves embracing one's true self and aligning one's life with personal values and aspirations. Readers discover how authenticity becomes a guiding force in the pursuit of happiness.

Understanding Authenticity:

Our journey begins with an exploration of authenticity—what it means to live in alignment with one's true self. Readers gain insights into the importance of self-discovery and the impact of living authentically on overall well-being.

Reflecting on Personal Authenticity:
Practical exercises guide readers in reflecting on their own authenticity. By exploring personal values, beliefs, and aspirations, readers lay the foundation for a journey of self-discovery.

Connecting with Core Values: The Pillars of Authentic Living:

The chapter introduces the concept of core values—a set of fundamental principles that define one's authentic self. Readers explore how connecting with core values serves as a compass for making choices that resonate with their true nature.

Identifying Core Values:
Guided reflections lead readers in identifying and clarifying their core values. From personal integrity to meaningful relationships, readers cultivate a deeper understanding of the principles that guide their authentic living.

Living in Alignment: Authenticity in Action:

Our exploration extends to the practice of living in alignment with one's core values. Readers discover how intentional choices and actions that reflect personal values contribute to a sense of purpose, fulfillment, and authenticity.

Aligning Actions with Values:
Practical applications guide readers in aligning their actions with their core values. From daily decisions to long-term goals, readers develop a roadmap for living authentically and intentionally.

Navigating Challenges to Authenticity: Overcoming Barriers:

The chapter addresses common challenges to living authentically and provides strategies for overcoming barriers. Readers explore how self-awareness, resilience, and self-compassion play key roles in navigating obstacles on the journey toward authenticity.

Overcoming Authenticity Barriers:
Guided exercises lead readers in developing strategies for overcoming barriers to authenticity. From external expectations to internal doubts, readers cultivate resilience and self-compassion as tools for staying true to themselves.

Cultivating Self-Awareness: The Key to Authentic Living:

Our journey takes a reflective turn as we explore the role of self-awareness in authentic living. Readers discover how cultivating self-awareness—the ability to recognize and understand one's thoughts, emotions, and behaviors—serves as a foundation for authenticity.

Cultivating Self-Awareness Practices:
Practical applications guide readers in cultivating self-awareness through mindfulness practices and reflection. By developing a deeper understanding of themselves, readers enhance their capacity for authentic living.

Expressing Your Authentic Voice: Communicating with Integrity:

The chapter addresses the importance of expressing one's authentic voice in communication. Readers explore how effective and authentic communication contributes to genuine connections and relationships.

Authentic Communication Practices:
Guided reflections lead readers in practicing

authentic communication. From assertiveness to active listening, readers develop skills that allow them to express their true selves with integrity and clarity.

Embracing Imperfection: The Beauty of Being Human:

Our journey concludes with an exploration of the beauty of imperfection. Readers discover how embracing their flaws and vulnerabilities contributes to authenticity and a deeper connection with others.

Embracing Imperfections:
Guided exercises lead readers in embracing imperfections as a natural part of the human experience. By cultivating self-compassion and a positive self-image, readers foster an authentic acceptance of themselves.

In this chapter, readers embark on a journey to explore authenticity—a practice that involves embracing one's true self and aligning one's life with personal values. Practical applications and reflective exercises guide readers in connecting with their core values, aligning their actions with authenticity, and navigating challenges on the path toward a more genuine and fulfilling life.

HAPPINESS IS FREE

15. The Art of Surrender: Finding Peace in Letting Go:

Explore the concept of surrender and provide practical strategies for finding peace and well-being through the practice of letting go.

Approach:

Surrendering to the Flow of Life:

In this chapter, we delve into the art of surrender—a practice that involves letting go of the need for control and finding peace in accepting the flow of life. Readers explore the transformative power of surrender in fostering well-being and embracing the beauty of uncertainty.

Understanding Surrender:

Our journey begins with an exploration of surrender—what it means to release the grip of control and trust in the natural unfolding of life. Readers gain insights into the benefits of surrender for mental and emotional well-being.

Reflecting on Personal Perspectives on Control:

Practical exercises guide readers in reflecting on their own perspectives on control. By identifying areas where the need for control may create stress or resistance, readers set the stage for exploring the practice of surrender.

Letting Go of the Illusion of Control: The Liberation of Surrender:

The chapter introduces the concept of letting go of the illusion of control. Readers explore how the desire for control can create stress and anxiety, and they discover the liberation that comes with surrendering to the inherent uncertainties of life.

Practicing Letting Go:

Guided reflections lead readers in practicing the art of letting go. Through mindfulness exercises and acceptance practices, readers cultivate a mindset that embraces the present moment without the burden of excessive control.

Cultivating Trust in the Process: Surrendering with Faith:

Our exploration extends to the practice of cultivating trust in the process of life. Readers discover how surrendering with faith in the unfolding journey fosters a sense of peace, resilience, and openness to new possibilities.

Cultivating Trust Exercises:

Practical applications guide readers in cultivating trust through exercises that encourage faith in the process of life. From affirmations to visualization, readers develop tools for surrendering with a sense of trust and openness.

Surrendering to the Present Moment: Mindful Acceptance:

The chapter addresses the importance of surrendering to the present moment through mindful acceptance. Readers explore how the practice of mindfulness enhances the ability to be fully present and engaged with the experiences of life.

Mindful Acceptance Practices:

Guided exercises lead readers in practicing mindful acceptance. From breath awareness to sensory mindfulness, readers cultivate a presence that allows them to surrender to the richness of each moment.

Embracing Impermanence: Surrendering to the Nature of Change:

Our journey takes a reflective turn as we explore the concept of impermanence. Readers discover how embracing the transience of life and surrendering to the nature of change can lead to a profound sense of peace and freedom.

Reflecting on Impermanence:

Practical applications guide readers in reflecting on the nature of impermanence. By embracing the idea that change is an inherent part of life, readers cultivate a mindset that allows for greater ease and adaptability.

Surrendering for Emotional Well-being: Letting Go of Emotional Baggage:

The chapter addresses the practice of surrender for emotional well-being. Readers explore how letting go of emotional baggage, such as resentment and grudges, contributes to a lighter and more joyful existence.

Letting Go of Emotional Baggage Exercises:

Guided reflections lead readers in letting go of emotional baggage through forgiveness and release practices. By freeing themselves from emotional burdens, readers create space for emotional well-being and peace.

Surrendering for Spiritual Growth: The Path to Inner Wisdom:

Our journey concludes with an exploration of surrender as a path to spiritual growth. Readers discover how surrendering to the mysteries of life and connecting with inner wisdom can lead to a deeper sense of purpose and fulfillment.

Spiritual Surrender Practices:

Practical applications guide readers in practices that foster spiritual surrender. From meditation to contemplation, readers cultivate a connection with their inner selves, leading to a profound sense of spiritual growth and fulfillment.

In this chapter, readers explore the transformative practice of surrender—a journey of letting go, embracing the flow of life, and finding peace in the present moment. Practical applications and reflective exercises guide readers in releasing the need for excessive control, cultivating trust, and surrendering to the beauty of impermanence for enhanced well-being.

16. The Wisdom of Reflection: Cultivating Insight for a Fulfilling Life:

Explore the power of reflection and provide practical strategies for cultivating insight, self-awareness, and wisdom in the pursuit of a fulfilling life.

Approach:

The Reflective Mind: Tapping into Inner Wisdom:

In this chapter, we delve into the wisdom of reflection—a practice that involves contemplation, self-inquiry, and the cultivation of insight. Readers explore how intentional reflection becomes a powerful tool for gaining clarity, self-awareness, and wisdom on the journey toward a fulfilling life.

Understanding the Power of Reflection:

Our journey begins with an exploration of the transformative power of reflection. Readers gain insights into how intentional reflection enhances self-awareness, deepens understanding, and provides a foundation for making informed and purposeful choices.

Reflecting on the Benefits of Reflection:
Practical exercises guide readers in reflecting on the potential benefits of incorporating intentional reflection into their lives. By identifying areas for exploration and growth, readers set the stage for the practice of reflection.

Cultivating a Reflective Mindset: The Art of Contemplation:

The chapter introduces the concept of cultivating a reflective mindset through the art of contemplation. Readers explore how contemplative practices and intentional thinking contribute to clarity, discernment, and a deeper understanding of oneself.

Cultivating Contemplative Practices:
Guided reflections lead readers in cultivating a reflective mindset through practices such as meditation, journaling, and mindful contemplation. Readers develop tools for incorporating contemplation into their daily lives.

Reflective Self-Inquiry: Asking the Right Questions:

Our exploration extends to the practice of reflective self-inquiry. Readers discover how asking the right questions becomes a catalyst for self-discovery, leading to greater clarity on values, goals, and the path toward a fulfilling life.

Reflective Questioning Exercises:
Practical applications guide readers in engaging in reflective self-inquiry through targeted questioning. From exploring personal values to envisioning future aspirations, readers gain insights into their inner selves.

The Wisdom of Past Experiences: Learning and Growth:

The chapter addresses the wisdom that can be gained from reflecting on past experiences. Readers explore how reviewing and learning from the past contributes to personal growth, resilience, and the ability to navigate future challenges.

Reflecting on Past Experiences:
Guided exercises lead readers in reflecting on significant past experiences. By extracting lessons, recognizing patterns, and acknowledging growth, readers harness the wisdom embedded in their life journeys.

Present-Moment Reflection: The Power of Awareness:

Our journey takes a mindful turn as we explore the power of reflection in the present moment. Readers discover how cultivating awareness through reflection enhances the quality of experiences, relationships, and overall well-being.

Mindful Reflection Practices:
Practical applications guide readers in incorporating mindfulness into reflective practices. From moment-to-moment awareness to reflective pauses, readers develop a capacity for present-moment reflection that enriches their daily lives.

Reflecting on Core Values: Aligning Actions with Beliefs:

The chapter addresses the importance of reflecting on core values and aligning actions with beliefs. Readers explore how intentional reflection on values contributes to a sense of purpose, authenticity, and fulfillment.

Aligning Actions with Values Exercises:
Guided reflections lead readers in reflecting on core values and aligning their actions with their beliefs. By making intentional choices in alignment with values, readers create a meaningful and purposeful life.

Wisdom in Decision-Making: Reflective Choices:

Our journey concludes with an exploration of the role of reflection in decision-making. Readers discover how intentional reflection becomes a guide for making choices that align with personal values, goals, and the pursuit of a fulfilling life.

Reflective Decision-Making Practices:
Practical applications guide readers in incorporating reflection into their decision-making processes. From weighing options to considering long-term

consequences, readers develop a reflective approach to making choices that contribute to a fulfilling life.

In this chapter, readers explore the wisdom of reflection—a practice that involves contemplation, self-inquiry, and the cultivation of insight. Practical applications and reflective exercises guide readers in developing a reflective mindset, engaging in self-inquiry, and harnessing the wisdom embedded in past experiences, values, and decision-making processes for a more fulfilling life.

17. The Art of Mindful Living: Cultivating Presence in Everyday Moments:

Explore the practice of mindful living and provide practical strategies for cultivating presence, awareness, and a sense of peace in everyday moments.

Approach:

Embarking on the Mindful Journey:

The Essence of Presence:

In this chapter, we delve into the art of mindful living—a practice that involves cultivating presence, awareness, and a sense of peace in everyday moments. Readers explore how mindfulness becomes a transformative tool for enhancing the quality of life and fostering a deeper connection to the present.

Understanding Mindful Living:

Our journey begins with an exploration of mindful living—what it means to be fully present and engaged in the current moment. Readers gain insights into the benefits of mindfulness for mental clarity, emotional well-being, and overall life satisfaction.

Reflecting on the Benefits of Mindfulness: Practical exercises guide readers in reflecting on the potential benefits of incorporating mindfulness into their lives. By identifying areas for increased presence and awareness, readers set the stage for the practice of mindful living.

Cultivating Mindful Presence: The Art of Being:

The chapter introduces the concept of cultivating mindful presence—the art of being fully present in each moment. Readers explore how intentional attention to the present enhances the richness of experiences and deepens connections with oneself and the world.

Cultivating Mindful Presence Practices:
Guided reflections lead readers in cultivating mindful presence through practices such as breath awareness, sensory mindfulness, and mindful observation. Readers develop tools for incorporating mindfulness into their daily lives.

Mindfulness in Daily Activities: A Path to Grounded Living:

Our exploration extends to the practice of mindfulness in daily activities. Readers discover how bringing present-moment awareness to routine tasks transforms ordinary moments into opportunities for connection, appreciation, and grounding.

Mindful Daily Activities:
Practical applications guide readers in incorporating mindfulness into various daily activities. From mindful eating to mindful

walking, readers develop a habit of infusing ordinary tasks with intentional presence and awareness.

Mindful Communication: Fostering Connection and Understanding:

The chapter addresses the importance of mindful communication in fostering genuine connections with others. Readers explore how practicing mindful communication enhances clarity, empathy, and meaningful interactions in relationships.

Mindful Communication Practices:
Guided exercises lead readers in practicing mindful communication. From active listening to mindful speaking, readers develop skills that promote understanding, empathy, and harmonious relationships.

Mindfulness for Stress Reduction: Finding Calm Amidst Chaos:

Our journey takes a practical turn as we explore mindfulness as a tool for stress reduction. Readers discover how mindfulness practices can be effective in managing stress, promoting relaxation, and cultivating a sense of calm amidst life's challenges.

Mindfulness for Stress Reduction Techniques:
Practical applications guide readers in incorporating mindfulness techniques for stress reduction. From mindful breathing to body scan meditations, readers develop a toolkit for navigating stress with greater ease.

Cultivating Gratitude through Mindfulness: The Joy of Appreciation:

The chapter addresses the intersection of mindfulness and gratitude. Readers explore how cultivating gratitude through mindful awareness enhances appreciation for the present moment and contributes to overall well-being.

Cultivating Gratitude Mindfully:
Guided reflections lead readers in cultivating gratitude through mindfulness. From gratitude journaling to mindful gratitude walks, readers develop practices that deepen their appreciation for the abundance in their lives.

Mindful Reflection: Nurturing Inner Wisdom:

Our journey concludes with an exploration of mindful reflection—a practice that involves contemplative awareness and self-inquiry. Readers discover how mindfulness enhances the capacity for reflective thinking, leading to greater self-awareness and wisdom.

Mindful Reflection Practices:
Practical applications guide readers in incorporating mindfulness into reflective

practices. From mindful self-inquiry to silent contemplation, readers develop a holistic approach that nurtures inner wisdom and self-discovery.

In this chapter, readers explore the art of mindful living—a practice that involves cultivating presence, awareness, and a sense of peace in everyday moments. Practical applications and reflective exercises guide readers in developing a mindful presence, incorporating mindfulness into daily activities and communication, and using mindfulness as a tool for stress reduction and gratitude cultivation.

18. The Art of Connection: Building Meaningful Relationships:

Explore the importance of meaningful connections and provide practical strategies for building and nurturing authentic relationships.

Approach:

The Power of Connection: Nurturing Meaningful Relationships:

In this chapter, we delve into the art of connection—a practice that involves building and nurturing meaningful relationships with others. Readers explore the transformative power of authentic connections in contributing to overall well-being, fulfillment, and a sense of belonging.

Understanding the Importance of Connection:

Our journey begins with an exploration of the significance of connection in human lives. Readers gain insights into the benefits of meaningful relationships for emotional well-being, personal growth, and a sense of community.

Reflecting on the Impact of Connection:
Practical exercises guide readers in reflecting on the impact of connection on their lives. By identifying areas for improvement and exploration, readers set the stage for the practice of building meaningful relationships.

Cultivating Authentic Connections: The Heart of Meaningful Relationships:

The chapter introduces the concept of cultivating authentic connections—the essence of building meaningful relationships. Readers explore how authenticity, vulnerability, and mutual understanding form the foundation of genuine and lasting connections.

Cultivating Authentic Connections Practices:
Guided reflections lead readers in cultivating authentic connections through practices such as active listening, vulnerability sharing, and empathetic communication. Readers develop tools for building relationships based on openness and authenticity.

The Art of Active Listening: Fostering Understanding:

Our exploration extends to the practice of active listening—a key skill in building meaningful connections. Readers discover how the art of listening with intention and presence enhances understanding, empathy, and the quality of relationships.

Active Listening Techniques:
Practical applications guide readers in honing their active listening skills. From paraphrasing to reflective listening, readers develop habits that foster deeper connections through mindful engagement.

Expressing Empathy: Connecting Through Understanding:

The chapter addresses the importance of expressing empathy in building meaningful relationships. Readers explore how understanding and acknowledging the emotions of others contribute to a sense of connection and support.

Expressing Empathy Practices:
Guided exercises lead readers in practicing expressions of empathy. From validating emotions to offering empathetic responses, readers develop the ability to connect with others on a deeper emotional level.

Building Positive Communication Habits: The Foundation of Connection:

Our journey takes a practical turn as we explore positive communication habits in relationship-building. Readers discover how intentional and constructive communication contributes to a positive and supportive relational environment.

Building Positive Communication Habits: Practical applications guide readers in developing positive communication habits. From using "I" statements to practicing assertiveness, readers create a foundation for healthy and effective communication in their relationships.

Navigating Conflict with Compassion: The Art of Resolution:

The chapter addresses the inevitable presence of conflicts in relationships and provides strategies for navigating them with compassion. Readers explore how conflict resolution can strengthen relationships and foster mutual understanding.

Conflict Resolution Techniques:
Guided reflections lead readers in exploring effective conflict resolution techniques. From active problem-solving to practicing compromise, readers develop skills that contribute to resolution and harmony in their relationships.

Cultivating Meaningful Friendships: The Joy of Companionship:

Our exploration extends to the realm of meaningful friendships. Readers discover the importance of cultivating and nurturing friendships, exploring how companionship contributes to a sense of belonging, joy, and support.

Cultivating Meaningful Friendships Practices:

Practical applications guide readers in cultivating and nurturing meaningful friendships. From intentional bonding activities to regular check-ins, readers develop habits that contribute to the depth and longevity of their friendships.

Connection in Family Dynamics: Nurturing Bonds:

The chapter addresses the significance of connection within family dynamics. Readers explore how intentional efforts to nurture family bonds contribute to a supportive and loving familial environment.

Nurturing Family Bonds Practices:
Guided reflections lead readers in exploring practices for nurturing family bonds. From family traditions to open communication, readers develop strategies for fostering a sense of connection and unity within their families.

Reflecting on Relationship Patterns: Building Awareness for Growth:

Our journey concludes with an exploration of reflecting on relationship patterns. Readers discover how intentional reflection on relationship dynamics fosters self-awareness, growth, and the cultivation of healthier and more fulfilling connections.

Reflecting on Relationship Patterns Practices:
Practical applications guide readers in reflecting on relationship patterns. From identifying strengths to acknowledging areas for growth, readers develop insights that contribute to the ongoing enhancement of their relationships.

In this chapter, readers explore the art of connection—a practice that involves building and nurturing meaningful relationships. Practical applications and reflective exercises guide readers in cultivating authentic connections, honing active listening and empathy skills, fostering positive communication habits, and navigating conflicts with compassion. The chapter also explores the importance of meaningful friendships, connections within family dynamics, and the role of reflection in understanding and improving relationship patterns.

19. The Joy of Giving: Cultivating a Generous Heart:

Explore the practice of giving and provide practical strategies for cultivating a generous and compassionate heart.

Approach:

The Transformative Power of Giving:

In this chapter, we delve into the joy of giving—a practice that involves cultivating a generous and compassionate heart. Readers explore how acts of kindness, generosity, and philanthropy contribute not only to the well-being of others but also to the fulfillment and happiness of the giver.

Understanding the Joy of Giving:

Our journey begins with an exploration of the transformative power of giving. Readers gain insights into the benefits of cultivating a generous heart, including increased happiness, a sense of purpose, and the creation of positive social connections.

Reflecting on Personal Motivations for Giving:
Practical exercises guide readers in reflecting on their personal motivations for giving. By identifying values, passions, and areas of impact, readers set the stage for the practice of cultivating a generous heart.

The Art of Kindness: Small Acts, Big Impact:

The chapter introduces the concept of the art of kindness—a practice that involves engaging in small acts of kindness that have a positive impact on others. Readers discover how kindness becomes a powerful tool for creating a ripple effect of positivity in the world.

Cultivating the Art of Kindness Practices:
Guided reflections lead readers in cultivating the art of kindness through

practices such as random acts of kindness, intentional giving, and expressions of gratitude. Readers develop habits that contribute to a culture of generosity.

Philanthropy and Giving Back: Creating Lasting Impact:

Our exploration extends to the practice of philanthropy and giving back to the community. Readers discover how intentional efforts to contribute to causes and organizations create a lasting impact and foster a sense of social responsibility.

Cultivating Philanthropic Practices:
Practical applications guide readers in cultivating philanthropic practices. From volunteering time to making financial contributions, readers develop strategies for giving back to the community in ways that align with their values.

The Joy of Sharing: Fostering Connection through Sharing Experiences:

The chapter addresses the joy of sharing experiences with others. Readers explore how sharing brings people together, creates meaningful connections, and contributes to a sense of community and belonging.

Cultivating the Joy of Sharing Practices:
Guided reflections lead readers in cultivating the joy of sharing through practices such as communal activities, shared meals, and collaborative projects. Readers develop habits that foster a spirit of sharing and connection in their communities.

Generosity in Relationships: Nurturing Connections Through Giving:

Our journey takes a relational turn as we explore the role of generosity in interpersonal relationships. Readers discover how acts of generosity within relationships contribute to mutual well-being, understanding, and the cultivation of strong and supportive connections.

Cultivating Generosity in Relationships Practices:
Practical applications guide readers in cultivating generosity within relationships. From thoughtful gestures to expressions of appreciation, readers develop habits that contribute to the positive dynamics of their interpersonal connections.

The Joy of Mentorship: Inspiring Growth in Others:

The chapter addresses the joy of mentorship—a practice that involves inspiring growth and development in others. Readers explore how serving as a mentor or guide contributes not only to the well-being of the mentee but also to the fulfillment of the mentor.

Cultivating the Joy of Mentorship Practices:
Guided reflections lead readers in cultivating the joy of mentorship through practices such as mentorship programs, knowledge sharing, and supportive guidance. Readers develop skills for inspiring growth in others.

Creating a Culture of Giving: Impacting the World Around You:

Our exploration extends to the idea of creating a culture of giving in various spheres of life. Readers discover how intentional efforts to foster a culture of giving within communities, workplaces, and social networks contribute to positive social change.

Cultivating a Culture of Giving Practices:
Practical applications guide readers in cultivating a culture of giving within their spheres of influence. From organizing community initiatives to promoting a culture of support in the workplace, readers develop strategies for creating positive impact.

Reflecting on the Impact of Giving: Personal Growth and Fulfillment:

Our journey concludes with an exploration of reflecting on the impact of giving. Readers discover how intentional reflection on their giving practices contributes to personal growth, fulfillment, and a deeper understanding of the joy of generosity.

Reflecting on Giving Impact Practices:
Guided reflections lead readers in reflecting on the impact of their giving practices. From assessing the ripple effects of their actions to recognizing personal growth, readers gain

insights into the transformative power of a generous heart.

In this chapter, readers explore the joy of giving—a practice that involves cultivating a generous and compassionate heart. Practical applications and reflective exercises guide readers in cultivating the art of kindness, engaging in philanthropy, fostering generosity in relationships, and creating a culture of giving. The chapter also emphasizes the joy of sharing experiences, the impact of mentorship, and the transformative power of intentional reflection on giving practices.

20. The Path to Inner Peace: Navigating Life with Calm and Serenity:

Explore the concept of inner peace and provide practical strategies for navigating life with calm, serenity, and resilience.

Approach:

The Quest for Inner Peace:

In this chapter, we delve into the concept of inner peace—a state of calm and serenity that transcends external circumstances. Readers explore the transformative power of cultivating inner peace in navigating the complexities of life with resilience and a sense of tranquility.

Understanding Inner Peace:

Our journey begins with an exploration of the essence of inner peace. Readers gain insights into the benefits of cultivating a peaceful state of mind, including increased mental clarity, emotional balance, and the ability to navigate challenges with grace.

Reflecting on the Meaning of Inner Peace: Practical exercises guide readers in reflecting on the meaning of inner peace in their lives. By identifying areas for improvement and exploration, readers set the stage for the practice of cultivating a peaceful mindset.

Cultivating a Peaceful Mind: The Art of Mindfulness and Meditation:

The chapter introduces the concept of cultivating a peaceful mind through mindfulness and meditation. Readers explore how these practices become powerful tools for quieting the mind, reducing stress, and fostering a deep sense of inner calm.

Cultivating a Peaceful Mind Practices:
Guided reflections lead readers in cultivating a peaceful mind through mindfulness and meditation practices. From breath awareness to guided meditations, readers develop habits that contribute to mental tranquility.

Embracing Acceptance: Finding Peace in the Present Moment:

Our exploration extends to the practice of embracing acceptance—a key component of cultivating inner peace. Readers discover how letting go of resistance to the present moment and accepting things as they are contribute to a profound sense of peace.

Embracing Acceptance Practices:
Practical applications guide readers in embracing acceptance through practices such as radical acceptance and present-moment awareness. Readers develop tools for letting go of resistance and

finding peace in the unfolding of each moment.

Nurturing Self-Compassion: The Foundation of Inner Peace:

The chapter addresses the importance of nurturing self-compassion in the journey toward inner peace. Readers explore how treating oneself with kindness and understanding creates a foundation for resilience, well-being, and serenity.

Nurturing Self-Compassion Practices:
Guided exercises lead readers in nurturing self-compassion. From self-compassionate affirmations to self-care rituals, readers develop habits that foster a kind and supportive relationship with themselves.

The Role of Gratitude in Cultivating Inner Peace:

Our journey takes a grateful turn as we explore the role of gratitude in cultivating inner peace. Readers discover how cultivating a grateful mindset enhances the experience of serenity and contributes to overall well-being.

Cultivating Gratitude for Inner Peace Practices:
Practical applications guide readers in cultivating gratitude for inner peace. From gratitude journaling to gratitude meditation, readers develop practices that shift their focus toward appreciation and tranquility.

Mindful Living as a Path to Inner Peace: Bringing Presence to Daily Life:

The chapter addresses the connection between mindful living and inner peace. Readers explore how bringing mindful awareness to daily activities becomes a path to cultivating a peaceful and serene way of life.

Mindful Living Practices for Inner Peace:
Guided reflections lead readers in incorporating mindful living practices into their daily routines. From mindful breathing to mindful movement, readers develop a lifestyle that prioritizes presence and inner tranquility.

Resilience in the Face of Challenges: The Strength of Inner Peace:

Our exploration extends to the concept of resilience and its connection to inner peace. Readers discover how cultivating a peaceful mindset enhances the ability to navigate life's challenges with strength, adaptability, and grace.

Building Resilience for Inner Peace Practices:
Practical applications guide readers in building resilience for inner peace. From reframing challenges to developing a positive mindset, readers develop strategies for facing adversity with calm and serenity.

Creating a Peaceful Environment: The Outer Reflection of Inner Peace:

The chapter addresses the importance of creating a peaceful external environment as a reflection of inner peace. Readers explore how intentional efforts to cultivate a serene physical space contribute to overall well-being.

Creating a Peaceful Environment Practices:
Guided reflections lead readers in creating a peaceful environment through practices such as decluttering, organizing, and incorporating elements of nature. Readers develop strategies for fostering a calm and harmonious external space.

Reflecting on the Journey to Inner Peace: A Lifelong Practice:

Our journey concludes with an invitation for readers to reflect on their personal journey to inner peace. Readers are encouraged to see inner peace as a lifelong practice, a continual journey of self-discovery, growth, and the ongoing cultivation of a serene and tranquil mindset.

Reflecting on the Journey to Inner Peace Practices:
Guided reflections lead readers in reflecting on their journey to inner peace. From acknowledging progress to setting intentions for continued growth, readers gain insights into the transformative nature of their ongoing practice.

In this chapter, readers explore the concept of inner peace—a state of calm and serenity that transcends external circumstances. Practical applications and reflective exercises guide readers in cultivating a peaceful mind through mindfulness, meditation, acceptance, and self-compassion. The chapter also explores the role of gratitude, mindful living, resilience, and creating a peaceful environment as key components of the journey to inner peace.

21. The Dance of Balance: Navigating Work, Life, and Well-Being:

Explore the concept of work-life balance and provide practical strategies for navigating the complexities of work, personal life, and overall well-being.

Approach:

The Quest for Work-Life Harmony:

In this chapter, we delve into the dance of balance—a practice that involves navigating the intricate interplay between work, personal life, and overall well-being. Readers explore how finding harmony in these aspects of life contributes to fulfillment, satisfaction, and a sense of purpose.

Understanding Work-Life Balance:

Our journey begins with an exploration of the essence of work-life balance. Readers gain insights into the benefits of finding equilibrium between professional responsibilities and personal pursuits, including enhanced well-being, reduced stress, and improved overall satisfaction.

Reflecting on Personal Priorities:
Practical exercises guide readers in reflecting on their personal priorities and values. By identifying key areas of importance in work and personal life, readers set the stage for the practice of finding balance.

Cultivating Work-Life Harmony: The Art of Prioritization:

The chapter introduces the concept of cultivating work-life harmony through effective prioritization. Readers explore how intentional efforts to prioritize tasks, commitments, and personal well-being contribute to a balanced and fulfilling life.

Cultivating Work-Life Harmony Practices:
Guided reflections lead readers in cultivating work-life harmony through practices such as goal setting, time management, and boundary establishment. Readers develop habits that prioritize both professional and personal aspects of life.

Setting Boundaries: Creating Space for Well-Being:

Our exploration extends to the practice of setting boundaries—a key element in maintaining work-life balance. Readers discover how establishing clear boundaries in professional and personal spheres contributes to overall well-being and satisfaction.

Setting Boundaries Practices:
Practical applications guide readers in setting boundaries. From defining work hours to establishing technology-free zones, readers develop strategies for creating space

for personal well-being amidst professional responsibilities.

Mindful Work: Bringing Presence to Professional Life:

The chapter addresses the concept of mindful work and how bringing present-moment awareness to professional tasks enhances the quality of work and contributes to overall well-being.

Mindful Work Practices:
Guided reflections lead readers in incorporating mindful work practices into their daily routines. From mindful task management to mindful communication, readers develop a mindset that fosters presence and satisfaction in their professional lives.

Finding Passion and Purpose in Work: Aligning Career with Well-Being:

Our journey takes a purposeful turn as we explore the importance of finding passion and purpose in work. Readers discover how aligning career choices with personal values and interests contributes to a sense of fulfillment and overall well-being.

Finding Passion and Purpose in Work Practices:
Practical applications guide readers in exploring their passions and aligning their career choices with personal values. From career assessments to purpose-driven goal setting, readers develop strategies for finding meaning in their professional lives.

Nurturing Personal Well-Being: The Foundation of Work-Life Balance:

The chapter addresses the foundational role of personal well-being in the quest for work-life balance. Readers explore how intentional efforts to nurture physical, mental, and emotional well-being contribute to a resilient and harmonious life.

Nurturing Personal Well-Being Practices:
Guided exercises lead readers in nurturing personal well-being through practices such as self-care routines, healthy lifestyle choices, and stress management. Readers develop habits that prioritize their health and vitality.

Building Supportive Networks: The Role of Relationships in Balance:

Our exploration extends to the importance of building supportive networks in achieving work-life balance. Readers discover how cultivating positive relationships and seeking support contribute to resilience, satisfaction, and a sense of balance.

Building Supportive Networks Practices:
Practical applications guide readers in building supportive networks. From professional mentorship to personal friendships, readers develop strategies for fostering connections that contribute to overall well-being.

Flexible Approaches to Balance: Embracing Adaptability:

The chapter addresses the concept of flexible approaches to balance and the importance of embracing adaptability in the face of changing circumstances. Readers explore how being open to adjustments contributes to sustained harmony in work and personal life.

Flexible Approaches to Balance Practices: Guided reflections lead readers in embracing adaptability and flexible approaches to balance. From adjusting goals to reevaluating priorities, readers develop a mindset that accommodates the dynamic nature of work and personal life.

Reflecting on Balance: A Continuous Journey of Adjustment:

Our journey concludes with an invitation for readers to reflect on their personal journey of balance. Readers are encouraged to see work-life harmony as a continuous journey of adjustment, self-discovery, and the ongoing cultivation of a balanced and fulfilling life.

Reflecting on Balance Practices:
Guided reflections lead readers in reflecting on their journey of balance. From celebrating achievements to acknowledging areas for growth, readers gain insights into the ongoing process of achieving harmony in work and personal life.

In this chapter, readers explore the dance of balance—a practice that involves navigating the intricate interplay between work, personal life, and overall well-being. Practical applications and reflective exercises guide readers in cultivating work-life harmony, setting boundaries, bringing mindfulness to work, finding passion and purpose, nurturing personal well-being, and building supportive networks. The chapter emphasizes the importance of flexibility and adaptability in maintaining balance and invites readers to reflect on their continuous journey of adjustment and self-discovery.

22. The Art of Resilience: Bouncing Back from Life's Challenges:

Explore the concept of resilience and provide practical strategies for developing the ability to bounce back from life's challenges with strength, adaptability, and growth.

Approach:

The Essence of Resilience: Navigating Life's Ebb and Flow:

In this chapter, we delve into the art of resilience—a practice that involves developing the ability to navigate life's ebb and flow with strength, adaptability, and a mindset of growth. Readers explore how resilience becomes a transformative tool for facing challenges and emerging stronger on the other side.

Understanding Resilience:

Our journey begins with an exploration of the essence of resilience. Readers gain insights into the benefits of developing resilience, including increased mental toughness, adaptability, and the capacity to find meaning and growth in the face of adversity.

Reflecting on Personal Strengths:
Practical exercises guide readers in reflecting on their personal strengths and areas of resilience. By identifying past experiences of overcoming challenges, readers set the stage for the practice of developing resilience.

Cultivating a Resilient Mindset: The Power of Positive Thinking:

The chapter introduces the concept of cultivating a resilient mindset through positive thinking. Readers explore how reframing challenges, fostering optimism, and embracing a growth-oriented perspective contribute to the development of resilience.

Cultivating a Resilient Mindset Practices:
Guided reflections lead readers in cultivating a resilient mindset through practices such as positive affirmations, cognitive restructuring, and gratitude. Readers develop habits that promote a positive and adaptive approach to life's challenges.

Adapting to Change: The Heart of Resilience:

Our exploration extends to the practice of adapting to change—a key element in resilience. Readers discover how embracing change, developing flexibility, and adjusting to new circumstances contribute to the ability to bounce back from adversity.

Adapting to Change Practices:
Practical applications guide readers in

adapting to change. From embracing uncertainty to developing a growth mindset, readers develop strategies for navigating transitions and uncertainties with resilience.

Building Emotional Resilience: Nurturing Well-Being in Turbulent Times:

The chapter addresses the importance of building emotional resilience in the face of life's challenges. Readers explore how developing emotional intelligence, managing stress, and nurturing well-being contribute to a resilient and balanced life.

Building Emotional Resilience Practices:
Guided exercises lead readers in building emotional resilience through practices such as mindfulness, self-compassion, and stress management. Readers develop habits that enhance emotional well-being and resilience in turbulent times.

Navigating Setbacks: The Strength of Perseverance:

Our journey takes a determined turn as we explore the concept of navigating setbacks with perseverance. Readers discover how developing grit, maintaining focus on goals, and learning from setbacks contribute to the ability to overcome obstacles.

Navigating Setbacks Practices:
Practical applications guide readers in navigating setbacks with perseverance. From setting realistic goals to developing a resilience plan, readers develop strategies for overcoming challenges and staying focused on their aspirations.

Cultivating Social Support: The Role of Connections in Resilience:

The chapter addresses the significance of cultivating social support in the journey of resilience. Readers explore how building and maintaining positive connections contribute to the ability to bounce back from challenges with a sense of community.

Cultivating Social Support Practices:
Guided reflections lead readers in cultivating social support through practices such as building a support network, seeking help, and offering support to others. Readers develop strategies for fostering connections that contribute to overall resilience.

Learning from Adversity: Finding Growth in Challenges:

Our exploration extends to the concept of learning from adversity and finding growth in challenges. Readers discover how developing a reflective mindset, extracting lessons from experiences, and finding meaning contribute to resilience.

Learning from Adversity Practices:
Practical applications guide readers in learning from adversity. From reflective

journaling to extracting lessons from setbacks, readers develop a mindset that transforms challenges into opportunities for personal and spiritual growth.

Resilience in Professional Life: Navigating Career Challenges:

The chapter addresses the application of resilience in professional life. Readers explore how developing resilience contributes to navigating career challenges, overcoming setbacks, and fostering a positive and adaptive approach to work.

Resilience in Professional Life Practices:
Guided exercises lead readers in applying resilience in their professional lives. From developing a career resilience plan to managing work-related stress, readers develop strategies for thriving in their careers despite challenges.

Teaching Resilience to Future Generations: A Legacy of Strength:

Our journey concludes with an exploration of the importance of teaching resilience to future generations. Readers discover how modeling resilience, fostering positive attitudes, and providing support contribute to the development of resilient individuals and communities.

Teaching Resilience to Future Generations Practices:
Guided reflections lead readers in considering how they can contribute to the development of resilience in future generations. From mentoring to fostering a culture of growth, readers reflect on their role in passing on the legacy of strength.

In this chapter, readers explore the art of resilience—a practice that involves developing the ability to navigate life's challenges with strength, adaptability, and growth. Practical applications and reflective exercises guide readers in cultivating a resilient mindset, adapting to change, building emotional resilience, navigating setbacks, and finding growth in adversity. The chapter also addresses the application of resilience in professional life and emphasizes the importance of teaching resilience to future generations.

23. The Journey Within: Exploring Self-Discovery and Personal Growth:

Explore the concept of self-discovery and provide practical strategies for embarking on a journey of personal growth and transformation.

Approach:

Embarking on the Journey Within:

In this chapter, we delve into the concept of self-discovery—a transformative journey that involves exploring the depths of one's inner self and fostering personal growth. Readers explore the significance of self-awareness, authenticity, and continual learning in the pursuit of a meaningful and fulfilling life.

Understanding Self-Discovery:

Our journey begins with an exploration of the essence of self-discovery. Readers gain insights into the benefits of self-awareness, the importance of authenticity, and the transformative power of continual learning in the journey toward personal growth.

Reflecting on Personal Values and Beliefs: Practical exercises guide readers in reflecting on their personal values, beliefs, and aspirations. By exploring their innermost desires and motivations, readers set the stage for the practice of self-discovery.

Cultivating Self-Awareness: The Key to Personal Growth:

The chapter introduces the concept of cultivating self-awareness—a foundational element in the journey of self-discovery. Readers explore how deepening their understanding of thoughts, emotions, and behaviors contributes to personal growth and fulfillment.

Cultivating Self-Awareness Practices:
Guided reflections lead readers in cultivating self-awareness through practices such as mindfulness, journaling, and self-reflection. Readers develop habits that enhance their ability to understand and connect with their inner selves.

Authentic Living: Embracing Your True Self:

Our exploration extends to the practice of authentic living—the conscious choice to embrace and express one's true self. Readers discover how aligning actions with values, embracing vulnerability, and living authentically contribute to a sense of purpose and fulfillment.

Authentic Living Practices:
Practical applications guide readers in embracing authentic living. From practicing vulnerability to aligning actions with values, readers develop strategies for living in alignment with their true selves.

The Art of Self-Expression: Nurturing Creativity and Passion:

The chapter addresses the importance of self-expression in the journey of self-discovery. Readers explore how nurturing creativity, pursuing passions, and expressing themselves contribute to a richer and more authentic life.

The Art of Self-Expression Practices:
Guided exercises lead readers in exploring self-expression through practices such as creative pursuits, passion projects, and authentic communication. Readers develop habits that allow them to express their unique perspectives and talents.

Continual Learning: A Lifelong Journey of Growth:

Our journey takes an educational turn as we explore the concept of continual learning—a lifelong commitment to growth and development. Readers discover how embracing curiosity, seeking new experiences, and fostering a love for learning contribute to personal and intellectual growth.

Continual Learning Practices:
Practical applications guide readers in embracing continual learning. From setting learning goals to exploring new hobbies, readers develop strategies for cultivating a mindset of curiosity and ongoing growth.

Facing Challenges as Catalysts for Growth:

The chapter addresses the transformative power of facing challenges as catalysts for personal growth. Readers explore how reframing setbacks, learning from adversity, and viewing challenges as opportunities contribute to resilience and development.

Facing Challenges as Catalysts for Growth Practices:
Guided reflections lead readers in facing

challenges as catalysts for growth. From reframing perspectives to extracting lessons from setbacks, readers develop a mindset that transforms challenges into opportunities for personal evolution.

Building Healthy Habits: The Foundation of Well-Being:

Our exploration extends to the importance of building healthy habits in the journey of self-discovery. Readers discover how intentional efforts to cultivate positive habits contribute to overall well-being, energy, and a balanced and fulfilling life.

Building Healthy Habits Practices:
Practical applications guide readers in building healthy habits. From establishing a morning routine to prioritizing self-care, readers develop strategies for incorporating positive behaviors into their daily lives.

Exploring Spirituality: Finding Meaning and Connection:

The chapter addresses the exploration of spirituality as a dimension of self-discovery. Readers discover how seeking meaning, connecting with a sense of purpose, and exploring spiritual practices contribute to a deeper understanding of the self.

Exploring Spirituality Practices:
Guided exercises lead readers in exploring spirituality through practices such as meditation, prayer, or mindfulness. Readers develop habits that foster a sense of connection, purpose, and inner peace.

Reflecting on the Journey of Self-Discovery: A Continual Unfolding:

Our journey concludes with an invitation for readers to reflect on their personal journey of self-discovery. Readers are encouraged to see self-discovery as a continual unfolding—a journey of exploration, growth, and the ongoing discovery of the depths of their inner selves.

Reflecting on the Journey of Self-Discovery Practices:
Guided reflections lead readers in reflecting on their journey of self-discovery. From acknowledging personal growth to setting intentions for continued exploration, readers gain insights into the transformative nature of their ongoing journey.

In this chapter, readers explore the concept of self-discovery—a transformative journey that involves cultivating self-awareness, embracing authenticity, expressing creativity and passion, and committing to continual learning and growth. Practical applications and reflective exercises guide readers in the practices of self-awareness, authentic living, self-expression, continual learning, facing challenges, building healthy habits, exploring spirituality, and reflecting on the ongoing journey of self-discovery.

24. The Ripple Effect: Making a Positive Impact in the World:

Explore the concept of making a positive impact and provide practical strategies for contributing to the well-being of others and the world.

Approach:

The Power of Positive Impact:

In this chapter, we delve into the concept of making a positive impact—a practice that involves contributing to the well-being of others and the world. Readers explore how small acts of kindness, intentional efforts, and a sense of social responsibility create a ripple effect that can lead to positive change.

Understanding Positive Impact:

Our journey begins with an exploration of the essence of positive impact. Readers gain insights into the benefits of contributing to the well-being of others, fostering a sense of community, and creating a positive ripple effect in the world.

Reflecting on Personal Values and Social Responsibility:
Practical exercises guide readers in reflecting on their personal values and sense of social responsibility. By exploring their connection to the well-being of others and the world, readers set the stage for the practice of making a positive impact.

Acts of Kindness: The Ripple Effect in Action:

The chapter introduces the concept of acts of kindness as a powerful way to create a positive ripple effect. Readers discover how simple, intentional acts of kindness can have far-reaching impacts on individuals and communities.

Acts of Kindness Practices:
Guided reflections lead readers in

incorporating acts of kindness into their daily lives. From random acts of kindness to planned gestures, readers develop habits that contribute to the creation of a positive and compassionate world.

Volunteerism and Service: Contributing to Community Well-Being:

Our exploration extends to the practice of volunteerism and service as a means of contributing to community well-being. Readers discover how intentional efforts to give back to the community create positive impacts and foster a sense of social connection.

Volunteerism and Service Practices:
Practical applications guide readers in engaging in volunteerism and service. From finding local opportunities to contributing skills and expertise, readers develop

strategies for actively participating in the betterment of their communities.

Sustainable Living: Nurturing the Environment:

The chapter addresses the importance of sustainable living as a way to make a positive impact on the environment. Readers explore how conscious choices, eco-friendly practices, and a commitment to sustainability contribute to a healthier planet.

Sustainable Living Practices:
Guided exercises lead readers in adopting sustainable living practices. From reducing waste to supporting eco-friendly initiatives, readers develop habits that contribute to environmental conservation and a positive impact on the world.

Social Entrepreneurship: Innovating for Positive Change:

Our journey takes an entrepreneurial turn as we explore the concept of social entrepreneurship. Readers discover how innovative business models and ventures can be a powerful force for positive change, addressing social and environmental challenges.

Social Entrepreneurship Practices:
Practical applications guide readers in exploring social entrepreneurship. From developing social impact projects to supporting socially conscious businesses, readers develop strategies for contributing to positive change through entrepreneurial endeavors.

Advocacy and Awareness: Amplifying Voices for Change:

The chapter addresses the importance of advocacy and awareness as tools for making a positive impact on societal issues. Readers explore how raising awareness, advocating for change, and amplifying marginalized voices contribute to social progress.

Advocacy and Awareness Practices:
Guided reflections lead readers in engaging in advocacy and awareness efforts. From sharing information on social media to participating in advocacy campaigns, readers develop strategies for using their voices to create positive change.

Cultivating Empathy and Compassion: A Foundation for Positive Impact:

Our exploration extends to the cultivation of empathy and compassion as foundational elements for making a positive impact. Readers discover how understanding and connecting with the experiences of others contribute to compassionate actions and positive change.

Cultivating Empathy and Compassion Practices:
Practical applications guide readers in cultivating empathy and compassion. From actively listening to others' experiences to practicing empathy-building exercises, readers develop habits that foster a deep sense of understanding and connection.

Teaching the Next Generation: Fostering a Legacy of Goodness:

The chapter addresses the importance of teaching the next generation about making a positive impact. Readers explore how modeling positive behaviors, instilling values of kindness and compassion, and fostering a sense of social responsibility contribute to a legacy of goodness.

Teaching the Next Generation Practices:
Guided exercises lead readers in considering how they can contribute to the positive development of the next generation. From mentoring to promoting social awareness,

readers reflect on their role in passing on a legacy of positive impact.

Reflecting on a Life of Positive Impact: A Fulfilling Journey:

Our journey concludes with an invitation for readers to reflect on the impact they've made and the positive changes they've contributed to. Readers are encouraged to see a life of positive impact as a fulfilling journey—a continual effort to contribute to the well-being of others and the world.

Reflecting on a Life of Positive Impact Practices:
Guided reflections lead readers in reflecting on their journey of making a positive impact. From acknowledging contributions to setting intentions for continued efforts, readers gain insights into

Conclusion: Embracing a Life of Fulfillment and Well-Being

In this transformative journey through "The Essence of Happiness: Explore, Define, Live," we've embarked on a profound exploration of the fundamental nature of happiness and the myriad ways it intertwines with our lives. From redefining happiness to delving into the art of resilience, work-life balance, self-discovery, and making a positive impact, we've uncovered the keys to a fulfilling and well-lived life.

Reflecting on the Essence of Happiness:

Our journey began by challenging traditional definitions of happiness, urging readers to construct their own understanding. We explored fleeting emotions, sustained states of being, and the unique combination that defines happiness for each individual. Through thought-provoking exercises, readers contemplated the essence of their own happiness and embarked on a journey of self-discovery.

A Deep Dive into Defining Happiness:

The journey continued with a closer look at defining happiness. We engaged in exercises to uncover personal values, beliefs, and sources of joy. Readers explored the multi-faceted nature of happiness, recognizing its connection to purpose, relationships, and self-fulfillment. The chapter set the stage for a nuanced understanding that goes beyond fleeting pleasures.

Cultivating Inner Peace: The Foundation of Happiness:

The exploration deepened with a focus on cultivating inner peace—a cornerstone of true happiness. Readers discovered the transformative power of mindfulness, meditation, acceptance, and self-compassion. Practical applications guided them in creating a peaceful mindset, fostering resilience, and finding serenity in the present moment.

The Dance of Balance: Navigating Work, Life, and Well-Being:

The dance of balance took center stage as we explored the intricacies of work-life harmony. From effective prioritization and setting boundaries to mindful work practices and finding passion, readers gained insights into creating a fulfilling and balanced life. The chapter emphasized the role of personal well-being in achieving harmony and resilience in the face of challenges.

The Art of Resilience: Bouncing Back from Life's Challenges:

Resilience emerged as a transformative tool for navigating life's challenges. Readers learned to cultivate a resilient mindset, adapt to change, build emotional resilience, and navigate setbacks with perseverance. The chapter emphasized the importance of embracing adversity as an opportunity for growth and developing resilience in both personal and professional spheres.

The Journey Within: Exploring Self-Discovery and Personal Growth:

The journey within took us on a path of self-discovery and personal growth. Readers explored the significance of self-awareness, authentic living, self-expression, continual learning, and facing challenges as catalysts for development. The chapter encouraged the cultivation of healthy habits, the exploration of spirituality, and a continual unfolding of one's inner self.

The Ripple Effect: Making a Positive Impact in the World:

Our exploration concluded with the powerful concept of making a positive impact. Readers delved into acts of kindness, volunteerism, sustainable living, social entrepreneurship, advocacy, and the cultivation of empathy and compassion. The chapter emphasized the importance of teaching the next generation and reflected on the profound legacy that a life of positive impact creates.

A Lifelong Journey of Fulfillment:

As we reach the culmination of this exploration, it's essential to recognize that the pursuit of happiness is a lifelong journey. Happiness is not a destination but a continual process of self-discovery, growth, and contributing to the well-being of others. By embracing inner peace, balance, resilience, self-discovery, and positive impact, readers are empowered to create a life of fulfillment and well-being.

Set Your Intentions, Embrace the Journey:

As we conclude this journey, set your intentions for the path ahead. Embrace the lessons learned, the insights gained, and the transformations experienced. The essence of happiness lies not in a single moment but in the intentional choices we make every day. May your journey be filled with joy, purpose, and the fulfillment that comes from living a life true to yourself and positively impacting the world around you.

Thank you for joining this exploration of happiness and well-being. May your path be illuminated by the essence of happiness in all its beauty and complexity.